AF618542

Infectious Diseases of Animals

Infectious Diseases of Animals Their Identification & Treatment

by

Sukdeb Nandi & Vishal Chander

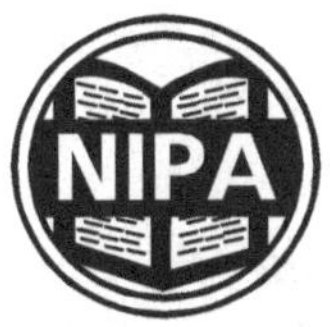

2012

New India Publishing Agency

Pitam Pura, New Delhi-110 088

Published by

Sumit Pal Jain for

New India Publishing Agency
101, Vikas Surya Plaza, CU Block, L.S.C. Mkt.,
Pitam Pura, New Delhi-110 088, (India)
Phone : 011-27341616, Fax : 011-27341717
Mobile : 09717133558
E-mail : info@nipabooks.com
Web : www.nipabooks.com

ISBN : 978-93-81450-39-0

Laser Type Setting and Printed at : Jai Bharat Printing Press, Delhi.-110032

CONTENTS

A. Viral Diseases

1

Foot and Mouth Disease

Synonyms : Aphthous fever; Contagious aptha; Panzootic aptha; Vesicular aptha.

Foot and mouth disease (FMD) is an acute, highly communicable viral disease affecting cloven hoofed animals, both domesticated and wild. It is the most contagious disease known in the animal kingdom. It is characterized by vesicular eruptions in the epithelium of the buccal cavity, tongue, nares, muzzle, feet, teats and udder.

Etiology : FMD was first demonstrated by Loeffler and Frosch that a filterable agent caused the disease and this was the first demonstration that a disease of animals was caused by a filterable agent and thus discovered the first vertebrates virus. FMD virus is under the genus *Aphthovirus* within the family *Picornaviridae*. It is a single stranded positive sense RNA virus with a protein coat consisting of four capsid proteins named as VP1, VP2, VP3 and VP4. Out of 4 polypeptides, VP1 is the most immunogenic one responsible for conferring protection in immunized animals. The icosahedral shaped FMD virus is about 23 nm in diameter with a molecular weight of $8.6X10^6$ daltons and consists of a single molecule of 8 kb RNA enclosed in a protein capsid. The genome of FMD virus is covalently linked to a small protein VPg at 5' terminus, an internal poly (C) tract and a poly (A) tail at its 3' end. The intact virion (146S particles) has a sedimentation co-efficient of 146S and degrades into 12S protein subunits when subjected to heat, low pH or low ionic strength. Empty capsids (75S particles) are devoid of RNA and contain 60 copies of each of VP1, VP3 and VP0 (the precursor of VP2 and VP4).

There are seven antigenically distinct types of FMD virus ; O, A, C, Asia-1 SAT-1, SAT-2 and SAT-3. The strains were named as 'O' and 'A' for Oise valley in France and Alemand in France respectively in 1922. In 1926 another strain could be demonstrated in Germany as 'C' strain. Strains designated as SAT-1, SAT-2 and SAT-3 were recognized from South African Territories during 1934 to 1948. Later, a strain could be isolated from Pakistan (South East Asia) in 1954 and was named as Asia-1. Unfortunately the virus seems to be capable of infinite mutation so that new antigenically different subtypes within each serotype are constantly appearing. There are more than 70 subtypes and within each subtype a large number of variants reported. The disease caused by the different serotypes is clinically indistinguishable, although the epidemiological patterns vary somewhat. The degree of difference between any two serotypes is such that an animal that has recovered from infection with one serotype is still fully susceptible to infection with other serotype. The difficulties presented to vaccination programs are obvious due to the presence of a large number of variants within each serotype as well as dramatic change in the virulence property. There may also be biotypical strains having the property to adapt to a particular species and infect other species only with difficulty. Thus there are strains that are virulent for pigs, some for cattle and some even for buffalo. Of the three standard strains, O appears to be the most common and C the least common. FMD has debilitating effects, including weight loss, decrease in milk production, and loss of draught power, resulting in a loss in productivity.

Susceptible hosts : Cattle, buffalo, sheep, goats and pigs are the main domesticated species infected. The water buffalo (*Bubalis bubalis*) can become infected and may also transmit infection to other species. Of all the species cattle are the most susceptible. Camelids, experimentally infected, contract the disease but do not transmit the disease to other domestic animals and play little or no role in the epidemiology of the disease. Young animals are severely affected than older animals and may die without any clinical signs. Secondary infections affect weak and debilitated animals.

Natural infection has been reported in many wild animals, including buffaloes (*Syncerus sp.* and *Bubalus sp.*), deer (Family *Cervidae*), impala (*Aepyceros melampus*), kudu (*Tragelaphus strepsiceros*), eland (*Taurotragus sp.*), wild pigs (*Sus scrofa*), tapirs (Family *Tapiridae*), reindeer (*Rangifer tarandus*), moose (*Alces alces*), American white colour peccary or javelina (*Tayassu tajacu*), coypu (*Myocastor coypus*), llama, alpaca and vicuna (Genus Lama), chamois (*Rupicapra rupicapra*) and antelope (Subfamily *Antilopinae*). The disease has been reported to occur naturally in European and African hedgehogs (*Erinaceus spp.*) and porcupines (*Hystrix sp.* and *Erethizon sp.*). The antibody to FMD virus has been detected in the tree and red kangaroos (*Macropus spp.*) and echidna (*Tachyglossus aculeatus*). Elephants, capybara and many rodents are susceptible and may provide reservoirs of infection for domestic animals. Suckling mice (*Mus musculus*, less than 14 days of age) are generally considered the most susceptible laboratory animal for research purpose. The guinea pig (*Cavia porcellus*) is also widely used in the laboratory but natural infection in this species and guinea pig to guinea pig does not occur. Rabbit and hamsters (*Cricetus auratus*) can be infected by inoculation but are less susceptible than guinea pigs.

There are very few scientifically authenticated cases of FMD infection in humans. It is not considered zoonotic. Human being exposed to infected animals can expel FMD virus through coughing, sneezing and breathing.

Distribution : Out of 7 serotypes, O, A and C have been identified in Europe and South America whilst O, A and Asia-1 are common throughout Asia. SAT-1 and SAT-2 are prevalent in entire Africa but SAT-3 is confined to Southern Africa. The strains found in Middle East include O, A, Asia-1 and SAT-1. Although some of the countries of the world like North America, U.K., Australia, New Zealand and Europe (except Southern Europe) have been successful to eradicate the disease, it is still enzootic in most areas of Asia, Africa, the Middle East and Northern part of South America. In 1546 Fracastorius described first FMD outbreak in Europe. Although South American countries Paragua and Argentina in 1997 declared "free from FMD with vaccination", it has been offset by the reappearance of disease in Malaysia, Philippines and Taiwan. FMD has been spreading north of Soviet Union from Iran, Afganistan and Turkey. In Europe, prophylactic vaccination has been ceased at the end of 1991 but there have been outbreaks of FMD in Italy in 1993, in Greece in 1994 and 1996. Outbreaks of FMD occurred in Bulgaria in 1991, 1993 and 1996, in Russia, close to Moscow in 1995, and in Albania, the Former Yugoslav Republic of Macedonia and the Former Republic of Yugoslavia (Kosvo) in 1996. Because the European part of Turkey, north of the Bosphorus (Turkish Thrace), is a part of Europe, it could be said that Europe has never been entirely free from FMD. In India the disease is recorded every year in almost every state of the country. FMD virus serotype 'O' has been found to be most prevalent (~88%) followed by Asia-1(~10%) and A (2%). The outbreak due to serotype 'C' has not been reported since 1998.

Mode of transmission : The disease is spread at an extremely high speed through direct contact with the infected animal or through infected fomites i.e food stuff, feeding utensil, water, cloth, harness, manger, beddings, straws, hay etc. The virus may occur in all the secretions and excretions of acutely infected animals. Airborne transmission is also an important mode of spreading the disease. The disease is first introduced to a new area via pigs which contract infection by ingestion of infected meat scraps. The disease is spread from pigs to cattle via movement of people, abattoir waste or animals mainly by oral route. Further spread the disease between cattle is by aerogenous route. There are peaks of spread at dawn and dusk. In pigs, the initial route of infection is by inhalation in which virus multiplies in the lung but disease spreads from pig to pig by the oral route.

In cattle, the first site of infection and multiplication of the virus is the pharynx. Subsequently, the virus appears in the blood and milk soon after infection and in the saliva before the appearance of vesicles in the mouth. All the secretions and excretions including the urine, milk, faeces and semen contain high concentrations of virus and may be infective even before the development of clinical symptoms and for a short period after signs have disappeared. The mouth and feet vesicles discharge large quantity of virus when they rupture. Affected animals are seldom infective for more than 4 days after the rupture of vesicles but virus may persist on the skin or hair. Some animals may remain as carriers for very long periods, and the intermittent passage of small amounts of virus may lead to the establishment of new outbreaks.

Carrier state in animals : The carrier state of FMD virus is an inapparent persistent infection in which intermittent recovery of virus from the oropharynx can be detected. The persistent infection in cattle and buffalo and to a lesser extent in sheep and goats, is a common sequel to both clinical and subclinical FMD. It is also established in vaccinated animals following contact with FMD virus, where virus replication is restricted to the oropharynx by protective level of circulating antibody. Carrier cattle are also defined as animals from which FMD virus is intermittently recovered in probang fluid after 28 days following infection. Titres of infectious virus in these samples, as determined by tissue culture, are invariably low and often fall below the level thought to be necessary for successful transmission to susceptible animals. Vaccinated and subclinically infected cattle can transmit infectious level of FMD virus to susceptible animals for up to 7 days P.I., whereas infection from true carrier cattle remains unproven under controlled conditions. Field evidence suggests that transmission occur from carrier buffalo to buffalo calves and cattle. Experimental infection of buffalo developed generalized infection and became virus carriers. During the acute phase of the disease in buffalo, the susceptible in contact cattle did not show any lesions, no virus was recovered and there was no development of neutralizing antibodies. However, cattle developed acute disease after 5 months and the nucleotide sequence analysis showed that viruses are identical to the virus inoculated to the buffaloes. So, it is inferred that in nature there is transmission of virus from buffalo to cattle, although there is little delay in the development of the disease without any change in the nucleotide sequences of the genome of virus during carrier period.

During the carrier period there is a gradual decline in the titre and frequency of virus recovery from the pharynx, which may be accompanied by any increase in non-infectious particles. The FMD virus RNA fragments have been detected in probang fluid samples after infectious virus can no longer be isolated. Despite reports of the seroconversion in calves following contact with carrier dams, transmission of FMD from carrier cattle to susceptible animals has not been shown under experimental condition. This may be due to the low virus titre in the oropharynx, cell association of persistent virus, presence of neutralizing antibody in secretory fluids, dilution and swallowing of secreted virus in saliva and altered virulence/infectivity of carrier virus. Treatment of carrier cattle with large doses of dexamethasone to reduce their immune response and allow amplification of virus in the pharynx had the opposite of the expected effect. All the traces of FMD virus disappeared from the pharynx and returned when the treatment was stopped. It might be due to the fact that dexamethasone induced immunosuppression caused the loss of virus along with disapprearance of the lymphoid cells from the pharynx. Carrier virus isolated from cattle was less cytopathic in cell culture than wild type virus and showed reduced virulence for susceptible cattle. However, the carrier virus retained its virulence for pigs and guinea pigs and regained its virulence for cattle after a single passage in pigs.

Site of predilection - The oropharynx particularly the soft palate is the predilection site for virus persistence in cattle although virus has been recovered from a number of organs and tissues for shorter periods during convalescence. However, the tonsillar region was found to be the site of virus persistence from where high titre virus could be recovered frequently. Virus could not be isolated from saliva suggesting the presence of cells and mucous in probang fluid is critical for virus recovery. The distribution of virus in the carrier sheep differed slightly from that found in cattle in that the high concentration of virus in the sheep was in the tonsillar area while in the cattle it was the dorsal surface of the soft palate and the pharynx. These difference might be due to the fact that in some sheep the tonsils project into the isthmus faucium to a greater extent than they do in the bovine.

Duration of carrier state - The duration of the carrier state is species related i.e cattle continue to excrete virus for up to 2.5 years P.I., sheep and goat for up to 9 months and African buffalo for at least 5 years. Strain variation also plays a role and affects the capacity of the virus to establish persistent infections. The carrier state is established both in vaccinated and non-vaccinated cattle following contact with FMD virus. However, the routine vaccination of cattle reduced the establishment of carrier in endemic areas, probably by reducing clinical cases and challenge doses of FMD virus.

Diagnosis of carrier animals - The identification of asymptomatic FMD virus replication is today equally important as the diagnosis of acute infections. The carrier animals may remain as the potential threat to other susceptible animals and may be responsible for secondary outbreaks. Such animals can be identified by isolation of virus from material obtained from OP fluids and by screening for antibodies to viral proteins which are not contained in the vaccines. Respective candidate antigens are the non-structural proteins. At least six of these can be distinguished and antibodies to most of them have been found in bovine hyperimmune sera. But, the objective would be to determine whether there are antibodies in bovine sera which specifically indicate a post infection state.

The immunodiffusion test in agarose gels is widely utilized for the identification of antibodies against virus infection associated antigen (VIAA or RNA polymerase) in animal sera. Due to low sensitivity of the test, a liquid phase competition indirect sandwich ELISA was developed to identify and quantify antibodies against FMD virus VIAA. Sera from convalescent cattle reacted specifically with the protein band identified as the non-structural antigens 3A, 3B, 2C, 3AB, 3ABC and VIAA in Western blot and found to be superior and accurate in detecting carrier animals. The latest development in the detection of carrier state in animals is the detection of antisense RNA by PCR in oesopharyngeal fluid samples collected anti-mortem and tissue samples obtained in PM. The PCR is more sensitive than standard virus isolation techniques and may be used for the rapid detection of FMD virus in specimens obtained during acute state of FMD as well as persistently infected animals.

Survival of FMD virus : FMD virus is acid, alkali and heat labile but can survive for long periods at neutral pH and under low temperature condition. FMD virus is inactivated within 48 hours in skeletal muscle at 4°C and pH <6. The pH changes in pork are less than mutton or beef. However, in lymph nodes, coagulated blood and bone marrow obtained from these same carcasses, the virus remain viable for 120 days at 4°C. The survival of FMD virus in milk is more stable than virus added to milk. The survival of FMD virus in the atmosphere is dependent on the relative humidity (RH). It has been reported that FMD virus showed maximum infectivity at 60% RH and above, while below 60% RH, infectivity is reduced and little or no infectivity at 20% or below RH. The minimum doses to infect cattle, sheep and pigs by air borne route have been presented in the table. In the most favourable condition, FMD virus can initiate infection 150 km away from the point of outbreak and possibly across expanses of sea. There are peaks of spread at dawn and dusk. It is known that FMD virus can be excreted in the semen of the bulls prior to the onset of clinical signs and at titres of up to log 6.2 mouse ID_{50}/ml. Spread is therefore possible through the use of infected semen or through the activities of the AI operators.

As FMD virus is a naked virus without envelope, it is resistant to alcohol, ether and chloroform. Commonly used disinfectants do not have any detrimental effect on the virus. Sodium hydroxide or formalin (1-2%), sodium carbonate (4%) destroy the virus within few minutes. Tongue epithelium and morbid materials (lymph node and spleen) should be collected in 50% glycerine phosphate buffer, pH 7.6 for isolation of virus and diagnostic purposes.

Survival times of FMD virus in common fomites

Materials	Period
Wool	14 days
Cow and buffalo's hair	4-6 weeks
House flies	10 weeks
Foot wear	11-14 weeks
Hay, straw, feed etc	15 weeks

Survival times of tissue culture FMD virus in different pH

pH	Period
4	<15 sec
6	2 min
7	several weeks
9	1 week
10	14 hours
12.5	<15 sec

Survival times of FMD virus in simple media at different temperature

Temp.	Period
-5°C	1 year
4°C	4 months
37°C	1 day
50°C	1 hour
60°C	5 sec

Survival times of FMD virus in milk

pH	Temp.	Period
4.0	4°C	2 min
7.0	4°C	15 days
7.0	72°C	40 sec
7.0	80°C	<5 sec

Minimum doses of FMD virus to infect animals

Species	Respiratory route	Oral route	By insemination
Cattle	12	$1X10^6$	$2.3X10^3$
Pigs	20	$8X10^3$	NA
Sheep	10	ND	NA

Period of excretion of FMD virus relative to the onset of clinical signs

Source	Time (days)
Saliva	-10 to +9
Airborne	-1 to +4
Milk	-4 to +4
Semen	-4 to +7
Faeces/urine	-1 to +6
Lesions	0 to +11

Pathogenesis : Following entry, the FMD virus settles in the cells of the dorsal surface of the soft palate and lateral wall of the pharynx without producing any lesions in these sites. The FMD virus shows a predilection for the epithelium of the mouth, feet and to a less extent teat and characteristic lesions develop at these sites after an incubation period of 1-21 (usually 3-8) days. From the primary lesions virus invade the lymph and enter the blood circulation and viraemia is produced. From the blood stream, virus go to the site of predilections i.e epithelium of mouth, dental pad, feet and udder and produce typical vesicles. The lesions used to heal up within a short span if it is not complicated by the secondary bacterial infections. Damage of feet may cause loss of horny covering followed by sloughing of hoofs and udder lesions leading to mastitis.

Clinical signs : Infection with FMD virus can result in a variety of disease manifestations, depending on the species on animal, the strain of the virus, the route of infection and general health of the host. The disease is not usually fatal. Morbidity is 100% but mortality is less in indigenous cattle and comparatively more in exotic and cross-bred cattle. The severity of infection depends on the strain, subtype, serotype of virus and immune status of the susceptible hosts.

The incubation period of the disease is 2-8 days under natural condition but it may extend to as long as 2-3 weeks. The disease is characterized by elevated temperature of 40-41.1°C and appearance of vesicles or erosions in the mucosa of the mouth, including tongue, lips, gums, pharynx and palate. There is abundant salivation, the saliva hanging in long, ropey strings and a characteristic smacking of the lips. The vesicles are thin walled and contain a thin straw coloured fluid. These rupture within 24 hours leaving a raw painful surface. The animals refuse to eat due to pain in the oral mucosa. Subsequently eroded surface is taken over by grey fibrinous covering. Finally, it turns to yellow or brown and the epithelium is restored. Concurrently with the oral lesions, vesicles appear on the feet particularly in the clefts and on the coronet. Rupture of the vesicles causes acute discomfort and animal is grossly lame, often recumbent, with a marked, painful swelling of the coronet. In severe case, there is shedding of the hooves. Vesicles may appear in the teat leading to mastitis and occlusion of teat canal. Abortion and subsequent infertility are common sequels. In rare instances, lesions may be found on other portions of the skin such as vulva or scrotum. Young animals die without exhibiting clinical manifestations. Some animals show signs of gastro-enteritis. Young calves are rather more susceptible than adults and die without showing any clinical manifestations. Lesions in the myocardium are most common in the fatal disease in young calves, lambs, piglets and kids. The lesions appear as small grayish foci of irregular size which may give myocardium a striped appearance (tiger heart). They usually die as a result of myocarditis and myocardial degeneration.

The disease is usually mild in sheep, goat and pigs but is important mainly because of the danger of transmission of the disease to cattle. Sheep rarely develop acute form of the disease but there is high mortality in lambs due to myocardial and skeletal muscle necrosis. An acute syndrome may also occur in goats and pigs, but it causes only mild disease in cattle after experimental inoculation. Experimentally, infected piglets often die without exhibiting any signs, death being due to myocarditis. In pigs, there is severe involvement of the feet causing lameness with appearance of few lesions of vesication.

Post FMD complexes : A sequel to FMD in cattle is a chronic syndrome of dyspnoea, anaemia, overgrowth of hair and lack of heat tolerance (panting), diabetes mellitus due to lesions in pituitary gland and endocrine system disturbances.

Pathology : The lesions of FMD are relatively mild except in mouth, feet and udder. The characteristic lesions comprise of vesicles and ulcers. Vesicular lesions become apparent when sufficient amount of fluids accumulate inside. The typical vesicle has a blanched covering and contains colourless or straw coloured fluid which turns cloudy due to secondary bacterial invasion. The lesions may be extensive and found in pharynx, eosophagus, fore stomachs and intestines.

Heart muscles show degenerative changes. There is grey or yellow foci or streaks in the myocardium which may give the myocardium a 'tiger heart' appearance. Changes may also be found in the pancreas, trachea and bronchi.

Diagnosis : The need to identify FMD is of paramount importance in disease free countries as well as countries where it occurs enzootically. A febrile animal showing lameness and salivation may be suspected for FMD. Differential diagnosis of FMD from the other diseases i.e. malignant catarrhal fever, mucosal disease, rinderpest should be made on the basis of laboratory tests and necropsies.

Differentiation of vesicular diseases in different hosts

Disease	Cattle	Pig	Sheep & goat	Horse
FMD	+	+	+	–
Vesicular stomatitis	+	+	+	+
Vesicular exanthema	–	+	–	–
Bluetongue	+	–	+	–

A range of laboratory tests are available. Although conventional tests like complement fixation test, agar gel precipitation test, fluorescent antibody test are still in use in small laboratories, well equipped central laboratories prefer to perform the highly sensitive recent techniques such as enzyme linked immunosorbent assay (ELISA) using monoclonal and polyclonal antibodies and radio-immunono assay (RIA). Besides plaque reduction neutralization, radial immunodiffusion and serum neutralization tests are available. If antigens are not detected in fresh material, then virus isolation can be attempted by inoculation of susceptible animals or tissue culture. The propagation of the virus in unweaned white mice by I/M and I/P route produces degenerative changes of skeletal muscles and can be detected by the I/D injection of fresh vesicular fluid into the plantar pads. Vesicles appear on the pads in 1-7 days and secondary vesicles in the mouth after 1-4 days. The inoculation of large animals i.e., cow, buffalo etc is made through intradermolingual route. The vesicles appear on the line of inoculation. This may be used to diagnose the disease from other vesicular diseases based on the different species susceptibilities of FMD, vesicular stomatitis and vesicular exanthema viruses.

The preferred cell cultures are primary calf thyroid and primary calf kidney cell cultures and BHK21 (baby hamster kidney) and IBRS-2 (swine kidney) cell lines. The virus neutralization test can be used to test the serum of convalescent or recovered animals for the presence of neutralizing antibodies. Virus in the tissue samples can be detected using sandwich ELISA or immunocapture ELISA or typing ELISA using rabbit hyperimmune serum and guinea pig hyperimmune serum against different serotypes of FMD virus as capture antibody and tracing antibody respectively. Serum samples are tested for antibody using a liquid phase blocking ELISA or solid phase blocking ELISA to test the level of antibody in vaccinated animals. The virus infection associated (VIA) antigen which is only produced in association with virus replication in the host following infection not in vaccinated animals can be detected by ELISA. It can be used to differentiate vaccinated animals from animals recovered from infection.

Most recently molecular biological techniques namely PCR based on the gene coding for VIA antigen and VP1 polypeptide of all the seven serotypes of FMD virus have been employed for the diagnosis of FMD and respective serotype respectively. Further, nucleic acid hybridization using serotype specific probes and nucleotide sequencing offer the ultra sensitive means for diagnosis of FMD.

Treatment : As FMD is a viral disease, there is no specific treatment. Symptomatic treatments may be provided depending on the clinical manifestations to affected animals. Antiseptic mouth wash with potassium permanganate, sodium carbonate, boric acid and glycerine may be applied on the mouth lesions. Antiseptic or antibiotic ointment may be given on foot and mammary tissue lesions similarly.

Vaccines and vaccinations : Although a number of new generation vaccines such as recombinant DNA vaccine, synthetic peptide vaccine, subunit vaccine, epitope vaccine and lastly DNA or gene vaccine have aroused the hope of preventing and controlling the disease in a better and efficient manner, most of the third generation vaccines suffer from measurable amount of drawbacks in spite of their induction of protective immune response. The protective immune response often has been elicited by these vaccines only in laboratory animals and not in domestic target animals. So, the cell culture based inactivated FMD vaccines are still popular around the world and are being used widely as immuno-prophylactic agents against FMD. In India several manufacturing companies are marketing the monovalent, bivalent, trivalent and tetravalent FMD vaccines using serotypes O, A, C and Asia-1. The virus is grown in BHK21 cell line followed by inactivation with either formaldehyde, acetyl ethyleneimine (AEI) or binary ethyleneimine (BEI) and adjuvanted with mineral oil, aluminium hydroxide or saponin. The FMD vaccines are also available in the market as combined vaccines along with H.S. or B.Q or both.

Hindrances in controlling FMD in India : There are a number of hindrances to control FMD in India. The most genuine point is the occurrence of FMD virus in 7 serotypes (O,A, C, Asia-1, SAT-1, 2 and 3), more than 70 subtypes and a large number of strains. Besides, extreme genetic and antigenic mutability makes the virus to evade the immune response exerted by the immune strain. However, molecular epidemiological studies carried out at IVRI have shown that the vaccine strain is quite well enough to provide protection against the field strains prevalent in India. The availability of the vaccine in India is not enough to cover all the susceptible livestock animals and often cattle are the only vaccinated species. The cost of the repeated vaccination is beyond the reach of the poor farmers. The occurrence of carrier animals and lack of diagnostic tests to detect them remains a bottleneck to prevent the dissemination of virus to susceptible animals. The disease picture has been complicated further due to involvement of wild animals and there is no vaccination programmes destined to them. Wild animals remain as a source of virus to neighbouring animals.

Lastly, there is no legislative control to prevent the movement of animals from one place to another and vigorous checking system while importing animals from disease prone countries.

Control : The control of the disease in India is difficult due to many factors such as economic constraints, environmental factors, the co-existence of wild and domestic hosts, the short period protection afforded by vaccines, the virus itself and the human element. However, many countries in the world have succeeded to achieve FMD free status by strict implementation of the following measures.

1. Large scale vaccination of susceptible animals with strict quarantine and slaughter of infected animals.
2. Stamping out policy where all the infected animals are slaughtered and the carcasses are either buried or burnt, should be imposed through legislation.
3. All straw, hay etc. having contact with suspected animals should be destroyed and the premises should be cleaned and disinfected.
4. Restriction of animal movement should be made through regulation.

5. Import of animals from disease free countries only.
6. Lime powder should be sprinkled around the animal houses.
7. Highly effective and efficient serosurveillance and monitoring of the disease in the field and subsequent reporting to the competent authority.
8. Animals should not be allowed to drink water from ponds/streams/ rivers etc. Infected animals may contaminate those sources.
9. Disease can be spread by persons moving around the village. Their movements should be restricted. If it is not practicable, people should scrub themselves and their belongings with soap and caustic soda.
10. In case of outbreak, healthy animals should be attended first and then the affected ones. On attending the sick animals, people should wash himself and his clothes with 4% sodium carbonate solution. Utensils used for collecting milk should also be cleaned with 4% sodium carbonate solution.
11. Calves should not be allowed to suckle affected mother and they should not be fed with milk from affected animals.

The above mentioned guidelines should be followed strictly in a country where the FMD is endemic which in turn would be a great help to control the FMD to a large extent. It is quite possible to control the disease as it happened in Europe. Prompt reporting system, compulsory vaccination, vigorous sanitary measures and appropriate quarantine system would give the solution to the problem. However, all the susceptible animals should be vaccinated with a potent and effective vaccine besides strict legislation on animal movement and animal import from disease prone countries. While vaccinating the animals wild and captive susceptible animals should also be brought under the immunization umbrella. The carrier animals which harbour the FMD virus without showing any clinical symptoms should not be neglected as they are the potential source of virus to the susceptible animals and responsible for disease outbreak. Lastly, the co-operation and help from all corners including researchers, scientist, extension workers, field veterinarians, and farmers are needed to make it a grand success and to eradicate such an important disease.

Further Reading

Barnet, P.V. and Cox, S.J. (1999). The role of small ruminants in the epidemiology and transmission of FMD. *Vet. J.* 158 : 6-13.

Barteling, S.J. and Vreeswijk, J. (1991). Developments in FMD vaccines. *Vaccine.* 9 : 75 –85.

Black, L., Francis, M.J., Rweyemamu, M.M., Umehara, O. and Boge, A. (1984). The relationship between serum antibody titres and protection from FMD in pigs after oil emulsion vaccination. *J. Biol. Stand.* 12 : 379-389.

Black, L., Nicholls, M.J., Rweyemamu, M.M., Ferrari, R. and Zunino, M.A. (1986). FMD vaccination : a multifactorial study of the influence of antigen dose and potentially competitive immunogens on the response of cattle of different ages. *Res. Vet. Sci.* 40 :303-307.

Blancou, J. (2002). History of control of FMD. *Comp. Immunol. Microbiol. Infect. Dis.* 25 (5-6) : 283-296.

Brocchi, E., De Diego, M.I., Berlinzani, A., Gamba, D. and De Simone, F. (1998). Diagnostic potential of MAb based ELISAs for antibodies to non-structural proteins of FMD to differentiate infection from vaccination. *Vet. Quarterly.* 20 (suppl 2) : 20-24.

Cox, S.J., Barnett, P.V., Dani, P. and Salt, J.S. (1999). Emergency vaccination of sheep against FMD : protection against disease and reduction in contact transmission. *Vaccine.* 17 : 1858-1868.

Davies, G. (2002). The foot and mouth disease (FMD) epidemic in the UK 2001. *Comp. Immunol. Microbiol. Infect. Dis.* 25 (5-6) : 331-341.

Doel, T.R. (1996). Natural and vaccine induced immunity to FMD : the prospects for improved vaccines. *Rev. Sci. Tech. Off. Int. Epiz.* 15(3) : 883-911.

Doel, T.R. (1999). Optimization of the immune response to FMD vaccine. *Vaccine.* 17 : 1767-1771.

Doel, T.R. and Pullen. L. (1990). International bank for FMD vaccine, stability studies with virus concentrates and vaccines prepared from them. *Vaccine.* 8 : 473-478.

Doel, T.R., Williams, L. and Barnett, P.V. (1994). Emergency vaccination against FMD : rate of development of immunity and its implication for the carrier state. *Vaccine.* 12 : 592-600.

Domingo, E., Baranowski, E. and Escarmis, S. (2002). Foot and mouth disease. *Comp. Immunol. Microbiol. Infect. Dis.* 25 (5-6) : 297-308.

Donaldson, A.I. (1987). Foot and mouth disease : principal features. *Irish Vet. J.* 41 : 325-327.

Howard, S.C. and Donnelly, C.A. (2000). The importance of immediate destruction in epidemics of FMD. *Res. Vet. Sci.* 69 : 189-196.

James, A.D. and Ellis, P.R. (1978). Benefit cost analysis in FMD control pogramme. *Br. Vet. J.* 134 : 47-52.

Kitching, R. P., Knowledge, N. J., Samuel, A. R. and Donaldson, A. I. 1989. Development of FMD virus strain characteristics – a review. *Trop. Anim. Hlth Prod.* 21 : 153-166.

Kitching, R.P. (1998). A recent history of FMD. J. *Comp. Path.* 118 :89-108.

Kitching, R.P. (1992). The application of biotechnology to the control of FMD virus. *Br. Vet. J.* 148 : 375-388.

Kitching, R.P. and Salt, J.S. (1995). The interference by maternally derived antibody with active immunization of farm animals against FMD. *Br. Vet. J.* 151 : 379-389.

Moonen, P. and Schrijver, R. (2000). Carriers of FMD virus : a review. *Vet. Quarterly.* 22(4) :193-197.

Nandi, S. (2004). Foot and mouth disease vaccines and vaccination. *Indian Farming.* 53 : 12 : 9-12.

Nandi, S. and Suresh, I. (2006). Foot and Mouth disease in pigs – a serious concern. *Indian Farming.* 56: 6 : 33-35.

Nandi, S. (2007). Improved protection by optimizing immune response to FMD vaccines. *Livestock Line.* 1:2: 9-13.

Nandi, S. (2007). Constraints in the control of foot and mouth disease in India. *Livestock Line.* 1:4:7-11.

Nandi, S., Dash, P.K., Manohar, M., Deshmukh, V.V. (2007). Emergency vaccination against FMD. *Livestock Line.* 1: 7 : 3-8.

Nandi, S., Dash, P.K., Manohar, M., Deshmukh, V.V. (2008). Vaccination against foot and mouth disease in the event of an outbreak. *Livestock Line.* 1: 9 : 5-7.

Nandi, S., Kumar, Manoj., Patra, M. K. and Nandi, D. (2009). Characteristics of an ideal foot and mouth disease vaccine. *Livestock Line.* 3(6): 9-12.

Nandi, S., Suryanarayana, V.V.S., Banumathi, N. and Sen, A.K. (1997). Biochemical characterization of foot and mouth disease virus A10 and A22 subtypes by PAGE and IEF. *Comp. Immunol. Microbiol. Infect. Dis.* 20:1: 95-99.

Nandi, S. (2010). Current status, epidemiology, diagnosis and control of FMD. Lead paper presented in Short Term Training Course on "Laboratory Diagnosis of Animal Diseases and Zoonoses" on 13.12.10 held at Indian Veterinary Research Institute Eastern Regional Station, Kolkata from December 7-20, 2010.

Nandi, S. and Sen, A.K. (1995). Analysis of immunogenicity of foot and mouth disease virus subtypes A10 and A22 by micro-serum neutralization test. *Indian Vet. Med. J.* 19:3: 221-224.

Nandi, S. and Sen, A.K. (1997). A note on growth characteristics and plaque morphology of foot and mouth disease virus A10 and A22 vaccine strains. *Indian Vet. Med. J.* 21: 45-47.

Nandi, S., Swain, P. and Chakraborty, G. (1996). Foot and mouth disease in wild animals. *Asian Livestock (FAO).* XXI: 1:2-5.

Nandi, S. and Maiti, S.K. (1994). Foot and mouth disease carrier state in buffaloes. *Asian Livestock (FAO).* XX :7: 76-77.

Pay, T.W.F. and Hingley, P.J. (1992). Foot and mouth disease vaccine potency tests in cattle : the relationship of antigen dose, serum neutralizing antibody response and protection from challenge. *Vaccine.* 10 : 699-706.

Salt, J.S. (1993). The carrier state in FMD : an immunological review. *Br. Vet. J.* 149 : 203-207.

Sugiura, K., Ogura, H., Ito, K., Ishikawa, K., Hoshino, K. and Sakamoto, K. (2001). Eradication of FMD in Japan. *Rev. Sci. Tech.* (O.I.E.). 20(3) : 701-713.

Toma, B., Moutou, F., Dufour, B. and Durand, B. (2002). Ring vaccination against FMD. *Comp. Immunol. Microbiol. Infect. Dis.* 25 (5-6) : 365-372.

Woodhouse, M.E.J., Haydon, D.T., Pearson, A. and Kitching, R.P. (1996). Failure of vaccination to prevent outbreaks of FMD. *Epid. Infect.* 116 : 363-371.

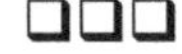

2

Classical Swine Fever

Synonyms : Hog eholera, European swine fever

It is an acute highly infectious viral septicaemia of swine of all ages characterized by rapid and sudden onset, high morbidity and mortality and generalized haemorrhages. A chronic course followed by recovery after treatment has been reported in older pigs and appearance of new born pigs with congenital defects.

Etiology : The etiological agent causing hog cholera is a linear single stranded positive sense RNA virus under the genus *Pestivirus* and family *Flaviviridae.* The virions are spherical, 40-50 nm in diameter and consist of a tightly adherent lipid bilayer envelope covered with glycoprotein peplomers surrounding an icosahedral capsid of 28-35 nm in diameter. The genome is 12 kb in length with 5'end capped but 3'end not polyadenylated. The genes for structural proteins are located at 5' end of genome. The virus replicates in the cytoplasm and matures within cytoplasmic vesicles. Though there is only one antigenic type of the virus, a number of strains of variable virulence and antigenicity has been reported. The causative agent was first thought to be a gram negative bacterium named *Salmonella cholera suis*. Later, it was confirmed that the disease is caused by a virus.

The most virulent virus strains produce clinical disease of pigs of all ages. The less virulent strains may produce little clinical disease primarily to fetal or new born pigs. This variation has occurred in the field strain of the virus but use of inadequately attenuated vaccine virus is also a contributory factor. The differences in variation in antigenicity and virulence have been recognized as a cause of vaccination failure and vaccine breakdown. It is closely related antigenically with Bovine viral diarrhoea virus (BVDV) and ovine Border disease virus (BDV).

Susceptible hosts : The pigs is the natural host for the virus and disease occurs naturally only in this species. All breeds, sex and ages of pigs are susceptible to this infection. There is considerable economic loss due to death of pigs and execution of control programmes. Experimentally rabbits and sheep have a low degree of susceptibility to virus. Limited transmission of the virus in goats, calves, cats and monkeys has been reported. Suckling white mice and rabbit are the most suitable laboratory animals for propagation of swine fever virus.

Distribution : The disease was first reported in Ohio in USA in 1833. Geographically, hog cholera has worldwide distribution. The disease has been eradicated from Canada, Australia, New Zealand and South Africa in 1918 and from U.K. in 1967. The disease has been reported in epidemic form in Federal Republic of Germany, the Netherlands, Belgium, France, Italy, Greece between 1982 to 1984. However, in 1985 six European countries namely Denmark, Ireland, Norway, Sweden, Finland and Switzerland have been reported to be free from the disease.

In India, the disease was reported in W.B. in 1951. Since then lot of outbreaks are reported throughout the year in different parts of the countries taking a heavy death toll and causing enormous economic losses which is aggravated further by high cost of vaccination programmes in enzootic areas.

Mode of transmission : It is a highly contagious disease and the infection is usually acquired by direct contact with infected pigs, ingestion or inhalation. Due to resistance and high infectivity, the virus may get access to the body through inert materials especially uncooked meat. All the secretions and excretions of the pigs infected with virulent swine fever virus contain virus including oronasal and lacrimal secretions, urine, feces, semen and tissue. Virus shedding can begin before the onset of clinical signs, and occurs throughout the course of acute or subclinical disease. Chronically or persistently infected pigs can shed virus continuously or intermittently for months. The virus continue to excrete in the urine for some days before clinical illness appears and for 2-3 weeks after clinical recovery. Disease transmission via the semen of infected boars may also occur.

In disease free areas, the disease is introduced through importation of infected pigs or the feeding of garbage containing uncooked pork scraps. Recovered pigs may act as carrier. Young pigs from non-immune sows infected with attenuated virus become carrier. In pregnant sows, the virus can cross the placental barrier to infect the foetus leading to still birth or piglets with congenital abnormalities. The virus may also be transmitted through insects, pigeon, flies, mosquitoes and human. Wild pigs act as inapparent carrier and transmit the disease to healthy domestic pigs. Transmission of the virus through egg of lung worm carried by earthworm which is eventually eaten by healthy pigs has been reported. It is also possible to transmit swine fever by grinding stable fly (*Stomoxys calcitrans*) exposed to infected pigs and injecting the materials into susceptible pigs. CSFV is moderately fragile in the environment; this virus is reported to survive for 3 days at 50°C and 7 to 15 days at 37°C. In refrigerated meat CSFV can remain infectious for nearly three months and in frozen meat for more than four years. This virus does not appear to be inactivated by smoking or salt curing in this proteinaceous environment.

Pathogenesis : The hog cholera virus is highly invasive and virulent. It apparently enters into the body through upper digestive tract or respiratory tract followed by septicaemia and invasion of vascular endothelium. The pathogen usually enters by oral route and the tonsils act as a primary site for viral replication beginning within several hours after infection. The virus then moves through lymphatic vessels and enters blood capillaries resulting in an initial viremia at around 24 hours. The virus multiplies rapidly in the blood and give rise to various clinico-pathological manifestations viz., fever, hyperaemia, inflammation, oedema of various organs and mucous membranes. There is degenerative changes in the endothelial cells which undergo swelling, proliferation and dilation and hyaline degeneration with infiltration of cells in the lumen of the wall of blood vessels.

In experimental infection, the disease is characterized by a biphasic temperature elevation at 2nd and 6th day P.I., a profound leucopenia and severe anaemia 24 hours after inoculation, diarrhea at 7th day and anorexia and death on 11th to 15th day. *Salmonella cholera suis* and *Pasteurella suiseptica* are the important secondary bacterial invaders to cause inflammatory changes in the intestinal mucosa and lung parenchyma respectively.

The experimental inoculation of pregnant sows with a low virulent field strain of hog cholera virus causes prenatal mortality in litters and post natal death when infected at 40 days and 65 days pregnancy respectively. Piglets of the infected sows may be born alive with immunological tolerance.

Clinical signs: The incubation period usually varies from 5-10 days although longer incubation period of 35 days or more are recorded. The disease may appear in three different forms viz., (a) Peracute (b) Acute and (c) Chronic.

(a) Peracute form

- It is most commonly noticed in young pigs.
- Young pigs die in about 24 hours without showing any clinical signs except high rise of temperature (106-107°F).

(b) Acute form

- There is high rise of body temperature (107°F). The peak of temperature rise usually occurs between 4th and 8th day of illness.
- Animals show dullness, depression, anorexia, vomition, constipation followed by diarrhea, dehydration and loss of body weight.
- Active hyperemia of the skin with purplish discoloration of snout,

ears, abdomen, inner side of the legs develops relatively early in the disease and is quite noticeable in the white hogs. A peculiar blotching effect on the ears may occur in acute infections but is more often seen in the more chronic cases. Small areas of necrosis are noticed on the edges of the ears, tail, lips and vulva.

- There are mucopurulent to purulent discharges from the eyes associated with conjunctivitis. In some instances a moderate to severe nasal discharge which subsequently may form crusts severely impending the passage, may be evident.
- Nervous signs comprising of circling, incoordination, muscle tremor, convulsion and paralysis are observed even in the early stages of the diseases. Death usually occurs 5-7 days after the initiation of illness. The infection with *Salmonella cholera suis* may aggravate the hog cholera disease result in high mortality.
- Reproductive disorders are observed when pregnant sows inadequately protected are exposed to virulent virus, vaccinated with live attenuated vaccines or exposed to low virulent field strains. There are mild pyrexia, high incidence of abortion, low litter size, stillbirths and abnormalities of piglets.

(c) Chronic form

- In chronic form mortality is 60-70% and morbidity is 90%.
- It occurs in the field outbreaks due to vaccination with serum virus mixture and characterized by prolonged incubation period, emaciation, alopecia, dermatitis, blotching of ears and abdominal skin. Recovery is usual after a brief period of illness but animals subsequently develop clinical disease and die in stress condition.
- There are signs of chronic diarrhea and chronic pneumonia.

Occurrence of clinical signs of hog cholera

Days	Clinical manifestations
1 to 6 days	High rise of temperature, leucopenia, decreased activity (slowness), conjunctivitis and piling.
4 to 8 days	Vomition, difficulty in respiration, convulsion, constipation and erythema.
6 to 20 days	Diarrhoea, incoordination, haemorrhages of skin, cyanosis of skin, blotching of ears and death in 4-8 days occurs in peracute cases, 9-19 days in acute cases and 30-95 in chronic cases respectively days.

Lesions

- Petechial and ecchymotic haemorrhages are noticeable under the capsule of the kidney, ileocaecal valve, cortical sinuses of the lymph node, bladder and larynx. In the early stages of the disease , the lymph node appear to be enlarged and oedematous. Parotid, submaxillary, cervical, bronchial, iliac and superficial inguinal lymph nodes show a diffuse type of haemorrhage. These nodes may be moderately red to almost black in color. All lymph node may show peripheral haemorrhage and described as mottled or strawberry like. Liver is dark, congested, swollen and shedds with mottled appearance. Petechial haemorrhages in the subscapular surface of the kidney may give rise to 'turkey egg' appearance. Lesions are found to be equally distributed in both kidneys. About 50% of the pigs suffering from acute or subacute hog cholera exhibit acute bronchopneumonia or congestion in the lungs.
- Spleen shows infarction due to disruption of blood flow and is considered almost pathognomic of hog cholera. The spleen becomes enlarged and darkened when congested. But congestion of spleen is most commonly found in salmonellosis and swine erysipelas. The gall bladder is frequently shrunken but in some cases is distended. Gall bladder shows infarction in the mucosa which is a common but not constant feature and appear to be almost pathognomic lesion. Thymic atrophy and depletion of lymphocytes in lymph nodes, tonsils and spleen are observed.
- The small intestine shows catarrhal enteritis, oedema, sloughing of mucosa and haemorrhage. Caecum and colon show 'button ulcer'- an encrusted, circular, raised lesion with concentric lines due to infarction of the intestine. This lesion is believed to be diagnostic of hog cholera. Later, secondary infection sets in and the circular lesion progressively becomes larger due to exuding mucous and cellular debris.
- Gross lesion of the brain are haemorrhages, congestion and oedema.
- An important antemortem laboratory examination is the total and differential count. There is pronounced leucopenia at the early stage of infection (total count reduced to 4000-9000/µl from 14,000-24,000/µl) and be a useful criterion differentiating it from bacterial septicaemia. In the late stages of infection, there is leukocytosis due to secondary bacterial invasion.
- Congenital infection leads to various foetal abnormalities and death of the foetus. Subcutaneous edema, hydrothorax and ascites is marked in stillborn pigs. Antibody is not detected in foetal blood when infection occurs early in foetal life. Hemorrhages occurs in the skin and many organs in the foetus.

Diagnosis: Prompt and quick diagnosis of swine fever is extremely important to avoid enormous economic losses due to high mortality in the herd. A confirmatory diagnosis is often difficult to make without laboratory examination as the signs and lesions of this disease are similar to that of swine erysipelas, septicaemic salmonellosis, pasteurellosis and streptococcosis. It would have been more complicated if African swine fever is present in that country since marked similarity of its lesions to those of hog cholera. The diagnosis is based on :

- History of an outbreak.
- Characteristic clinical symptoms.
- Pathognomic post mortem lesions- 'button ulcer' of the large intestine particularly in caecum, colon and ileocaecal junction and 'turkey egg' appearance of the kidney. Septicaemic, petechial or ecchymotic haemorrhages in the lymph node, epiglottis, larynx, urinary bladder, skin, lungs and thymus. Infarction in almost every organ especially in the spleen, gall bladder, lungs, heart, liver etc. Abnormal calcification of ribs at the costochondral junction near sternum of the growing pigs.
- Histopathological examination : Encephalitis is common feature in hog cholera infection. Brain tissue show vascular and perivascular infiltration with endothelial swelling. Acidophilic intranuclear inclusion bodies are seen in the reticular cells of lymph nodes, spleen and other organs.
- Animal inoculation tests : Groups of vaccinated and unvaccinated piglets are inoculated with spleen suspension of suspected pigs. Vaccinated piglets survive while unvaccinated piglets die showing characteristic symptoms of swine fever.
- AGPT : This test is designed to detect the presence of antigen in the pig tissues particularly in pancreas, lymph nodes, and spleen. Known antiserum is kept in the central well and the antigenic material in the peripheral wells followed by incubation at 37°C for 24 hours. There is development of precipitin bands in the positive cases and no band in the negative cases. This system has the advantage over the tissue culture system since it can be used for the detection of either antigen in the tissue or antibodies in the serum.
- HI test : can be employed for the diagnosis of hog cholera disease. In this test suspected test material is used as antigen and serum from recovered animals as antibody source. RBC is formalized and tanned. In the negative case there is agglutination of RBC and in positive case there is compact button formation.

- Fluorescent antibody technique : This test can be employed for the detection of intracellular swine fever virus from the infected organs i.e., tonsil, spleen, lymph node and the cell culture infected with swine fever virus.
- Neutralization test : Porcine kidney cell culture is commonly used for routine diagnosis of swine fever. This test is complex as this virus does not produce any CPE. Virus and different dilutions of serum are mixed and inoculated on to the monolayer of cells along with virus, serum and cell control. The presence of antibodies is detected by Fluorescent antibody technique.
- ELISA : This test allows the rapid, sensitive and specific detection of viral antigen in the tissues.
- Molecular biological techniques : Recently reverse transcriptase polymerase chain reaction (RT-PCR) using primers based on several structural protein and nonstructural protein genes allows the rapid, sensitive and accurate detection of viral genome in the tissues in a short period of time. Besides, nucleic acid hybridization, nucleic acid sequencing offer the detection of viral genome even in the tissue samples not suitable for other tests.
- Isolation of virus: The isolation of virus may be peroformed in pig cell lines sneh as rapidly dividing PK-15 cells. Cultures are examine by FAT after 24-72 hours or 4-5 days for immunoperoxidase staining. As a diagnostic tool, virus isolation is more sensitive than the direct immunofluorescence test (IFT) on frozen tissue sections.

Differential diagnosis

- Salmonellosis : The etiological agent is *Salmonella cholerae suis*. The infection is most common in pigs of 2-4 months of old whereas swine fever occurs in pigs of all ages. It causes several complications including diarrhea. 'Button ulcer' in swine fever is the result of exudation and cellular damage in response to secondary bacterial infection. The isolation of bacteria is needed to provide confirmatory diagnosis.
- Swine erysipelas : It is characterized by the peculiar diamond marking on the skin. In swine fever, kidneys appear as 'turkey egg' whereas in swine erysipelas the kidneys are congested and dark red in colour. It can be diagnosed by bacteriological examination and treated with antibodies.
- Coli bacillosis : It is caused by *E. coli* which produces disease during 1st week of life with high rise of temperature and death in 48 hours

due to toxaemia and dehydration. Gram staining of smears from faeces reveals Gram negative organism.

- African swine fever (ASF) : The disease is not prevalent in India. In ASF, button ulcer in the large intestine is not seen but necrosis of periportal hepatic cells are noticed. However, serological or molecular biological techniques should be carried out for confirmatory diagnosis.
- Streptococcal meningitis : The disease resembles with the nervous manifestations of swine fever. It affects pigs of 2-6 weeks of age. Gross lesions are not revealed. Diagnosis can be made on the basis of isolation of bacteria.
- Aujesky's disease : Young suckling piglets show convulsions and prostration due to nervous system involvement. The nervous symptoms are less pronounced in swine fever. Diagnosis can be made on the basis of serological test.

Treatment : There is no specific treatment of swine fever disease. Hyperimmune serum @ 50-150 ml/ animal may be of some value if administered at an early state of the disease. It has been proved useful in protecting in contact animals.

Control

- In hog cholera free areas: The slaughter of all incontact and infected pigs is generally practiced followed by burning or burial.
- All the vehicles, pens, premises and utensils must be disinfected with strong chemical disinfectants.
- Movement of the pigs should be restricted and in contact animals must not be sold in the market.
- Entry to and departure from infected premises must be controlled to avoid the spread of disease through footwear, garments etc.
- Boiling of all the garbage before offering as food to pigs should be practiced.
- Different persons should handle the affected and healthy pigs.
- In enzootic areas : Farmers should be educated about the highly infectious nature of the disease and the ease with which it can be spread by feeding uncooked garbage and purchase and sale of infected or in contact pigs.
- Routine vaccination of pigs with killed or attenuated virus should be carried out. Live attenuated virus vaccines produce a solid immunity and are capable of introducing infection and disease if vaccination break down occurs. Pigs vaccinated with live virus vaccines may show increased susceptibility to other diseases.

- In the event of an outbreak in herd, the in contact animals are administered with hyperimmune serum @ 50-100 ml depending on the body weight of the animal or immunized with vaccine. Pigs receiving only serum need to be vaccinated at a later date to build up a strong immunity.
- Adoption of suitable hygienic measures to prevent further spread of infection, disposal of carcasses by burning, isolation of infected animals and disinfection of pens are generally practiced.

Immunization : The immunity against hog cholera is classical example of the three major types of resistance to infection (a) Natural resistance (b) Passive acquired immunity (c) Active acquired immunity.

- Natural resistance to infection occurs on a genetic basis between species and within species. All the animals other than swine have strong natural resistance to hog cholera. About 5% of all swine are naturally immune to hog cholera disease.
- Passive acquired immunity : It can be obtained by two ways. (i) By injection of hyperimmune serum (ii) Passage of antibodies from the dam to the foetus through placental transfer or to new born through the colostrums.
- Active immunity is acquired by (i) Sublethal exposure (ii) Injection of an immunologically active form of the infectious agent by various ways.

Serum simultaneous method : In this method virus is injected @ 2 ml S/C followed by administration of serum which is produced by collecting blood 6-7 day after artificial infection in 20-75 ml doses depending on the size of pig to develop immediate, solid and long lasting immunity. Vaccination is carried out in pig of 4 weeks of age or more older. This method is not recommended now-a-days due to availability of safer vaccines.

Attenuated vaccines : These include attenuated strains by repeated passaging in tissue culture of porcine or other origin, lapinized vaccines produced by repeated rabbit passage and mutant strains. Many of these early vaccines were not stable and could produce disease, transmitted to in contact animals and produce foetal disease following vaccination of pregnant sows. Attenuated vaccines of Chinese or LPC and GPE strains origins are mostly used in Europe and Asia. They are antigenically stable and there is no evidence of reversion. They do not produce any clinical illness or leukemia. Immunity starts at 5-10 days. Piglets from nonimmune and immune sows should be vaccinated during first 2 weeks of life and at 2 months of age respectively. A cold adapted strain (French Thiverval strain) which has lost virulence but not antigenicity may confer protection from 5-10 days P.I. and last for 3 years.

Inactivated vaccines : These are usually prepared from the blood or tissues of infected pigs. Crystal violet and glycerin are added followed by incubation at 37°C to completely inactivate the virus infectivity. The vaccine was shown to protect pigs against both artificial and in contact animals and infection did not transmit the disease to susceptible animals and conferred immunity for ten months. Vaccinated sows may still develop fetal infection when exposed to virulent virus and the vaccine may induce virus carriers in endemic areas. Due to availability of better vaccines and presence of drawbacks, it is no longer used now-a-days.

Further Reading

Bouma, A., Stegeman, J.A., Engel, B., de Kluijver, E.P., Elbers, A.R. and de Jong, M.C. (2001). Evaluation of diagnostic tests for the detection of classical swine fever in the field without a gold standard. *J. Vet. Diagn.Invest.* 13 : 383–388.

Clavijo, A., Zhou,E.M., Vydelingum, S. and Heckert, R. (1998). Development and evaluation of a novel antigen capture assay for the detection of classical swine fever virus antigens. *Vet. Microbiol.* 60 : 155-168.

Colijn, E.O., Bloemraad, M. and Wensvoort, G. (1997). An improved ELISA for the detection of serum antibodies directed against classical swine fever virus. *Vet. Microbiol.* 59 : 15–25.

de Smit, A.J., Bouma, A., Terpstra, C. and van Oirschot, J.T. (1999).Transmission of classical swine fever virus by artificial insemination. *Vet. Microbiol.* 67: 239–249.

Dunne, H.W. (1975). Hog cholera. In. Dunne, H.W. and Leman,A.D (eds), Diseases of swine, 4th ed. Iowa: Iowa state university press, Ames, pp. 189-255.

Edwards, S., Moennig, V. and Wensvoort, G. (1991). The development of an international reference panel of monoclonal antibodies for the differentiation of hog cholera virus from other pestiviruses. *Vet. Microbiol.* 29 : 101–108.

Floegel-Niesmann, G. (2001). Classical swine fever (CSF) marker vaccine. Trial III. Evaluation of discriminatory ELISAs. *Vet. Microbiol.* 83: 121–136.

Gomez Villamendos, J.C., Ruiz Villamor, E., Salguero, F.J., Bautista, M.J., Carrasco, L., Sanchez, C., Quezada, M. and Sierra, M.A. (1998). Immunohistochemical and ultrastructural evidence of hog cholera virus infection of megakaryocytes in bone marrow and spleen. *J. Comp. Path.* 119 : 111-119.

Hoffmann, B., Beer, M., Schelp, C., Schirrmeier, H. and Depner, K. (2005). Validation of a real-time RT-PCR assay for sensitive and specific detection of classical swine fever. *J. Virol. Meth.* 130: 36–44.

Langedijk, J.P., Middel, W.G., Meloen, R.H., Kramps, J.A. and De Smit, J.A. (2001). Enzyme-linked immunosorbent assay using a virus type-specific peptide based on a subdomain of envelope protein E^{rns} for serologic diagnosis of pestivirus infections in swine. *J. Clin. Microbiol.* 39 : 906–912.

Mcgoldrick, A., Lowings, J.P., Ibata, G., Sands, J.J., Belak, S. and Paton, D.J. (1998). A novel approach to the detection of classical swine fever virus by RT-PCR with a fluorogenic probe (Taq Man). *J. Virol. Meth.* 72: 125–135.

Nandi, S. and Yadav, J.S. (2010). Classical swine fever – an alarming disease of swine industry. *Indian Farming.* 60: 9 : 28-31.

Nandi, S., Saha, S.K., Dandapat, S. and Samanta, S. (2009). Classical swine fever virus – its survival and inactivation. *Livestock Line.* 3 : 5: 12-14.

Paton, D.J., Mcgoldrick, A., Bensaude, E., Belak, S., Mittelholzer, C., Koenen, F., Vanderhallen, H., Greiser-Wilke, I., Scheibner, H., Stadejek, T., Hofmann ,M. and Thuer B. (2000). Classical swine fever virus: a second ring test to evaluate RT-PCR detection methods. *Vet. Microbiol.* **77**: 71–81.

Risatti, G., Holinka, L., Lu, Z., Kutish, G., Callahan, J. D., Nelson, W. M., Brea Tió, E. and Borca, M. V. (2005). Diagnostic evaluation of a real-time reverse transcriptase PCR assay for detection of classical swine fever virus. *J. Clin. Microbiol.* 43 (1) : 468–471.

Risatti, G.R., Callahan, J.D., Nelson, W.M. and Borca M.V. (2003). Rapid detection of classical swine fever virus by a portable real-time reverse transcriptase PCR assay. *J. Clin. Microbiol.* 41 (1): 500–505.

Vilcek, S., Stadejek, T., Ballagi-Pordany, A., Lowings, J.P., Paton, D.J. and Belak, S. (1996). Genetic variability of classical swine fever virus. *Virus. Res.* 43 : 137-147.

Wensvoort, G., Bloemraad, M. and Terpstra, C. (1988). An enzyme immunoassay employing monoclonal antibodies and detecting specifically antibodies to classical swine fever virus. *Vet. Microbiol.* **17 :** 129–140.

Wensvoort, G., Terpstra, C. and De Kluyver, E.P. (1989a). Characterization of porcine and some ruminant pestiviruses by cross-neutralisation. *Vet. Microbiol.* **20** : 291?- 306.

Wensvoort, G., Terpstra, C., Boonstra, J., Bloemraad, M. and Van Zaane, D. (1986). Production of monoclonal antibodies against swine fever virus and their use in laboratory diagnosis. *Vet. Microbiol.* 12 : 101–108.

Wensvoort, G., Terpstra, C., De Kluyver, E.P., Kraghten, C. and Warnaar, J.C. (1989b). Antigenic differentiation of pestivirus strains with monoclonal antibodies against hog cholera virus. *Vet. Microbiol.* 21 : 9–20.

Wirz, B., Tratschin, J,D., Muller, H.K. and Mitchell, D.B. (1993). Detection of hog cholera virus and differentiation from other pestiviruses by polymerase chain reaction. *J. Clin. Microbiol.* 31 : 1148-1154.

3

Rabies

Synonym : Hydrophobia, Lyssa, Jalatanka

This is an acute highly fatal viral disease of all warm blooded animals including man characterized by signs of abnormal behaviour, nervous symptoms (increased excitability and irritability), impairment of consciousness, ascending paralysis and death. The disease was variously known as lytta or lyssa coming from the belief that the disease was caused by a worm under the tongue (lytta) or hydrophobia, which describes the thirst and fear of water associated with the disease. The English name rabies derived from Latin word 'Rabere' which has been derived from Sanskrit word 'Rabhas' meaning raging, furious, savage, madness or to do violence whereas Greek term hydrophobia is now specifically used for rabies in man. The symptom hydrophobia (fear of water) is developed due to painful spasm of muscles of deglutition.

Distribution : The disease is known since ancient time. The disease has been recorded in various parts of the world in different species of animals. Australia, Britain, Scandinavian, New Zealand, Singapore, Hong Kong, Hawaii and some other Islands are free from rabies. This was possible due to strict quarantine measures and restriction on import of animal and animal products from disease prone areas. Lot of outbreaks are reported in India throughout the year causing 30,000 death annually and number of death toll may be higher as many cases go unnoticed. India accounts for the 80% casualties from rabies worldwide.

Etiology : Rabies is caused by a RNA virus belonging to the family *Rhabdoviridae* and genus *Lyssavirus*. It is a highly neurotropic virus and measures about 180-250 nm in length and 75 nm in diameter. The virus is bullet shaped and consist of a lipid containing bilayer envelope with glycoprotein peplomers surrounding a helical shaped nucleocapsid. It contains a single stranded linear molecule of negative sense RNA of 13-16 Kb in length which codes for 5 separate proteins. The virion possess a helical nucleocapsid core surrounded by an envelope of host cell origin. The genus lyssa virus contains classical rabies , Mokola, Lagosbat, Duvenhage, European bat lyssavirus 1 (EBL 1), European bat lyssavirus 2 (EBL 2) and Australian bat lyssa virus (ABL ; proposed genotype 7) under different genotypes. All the viruses except classical rabies virus are called rabies related viruses. All are capable of causing clinically indistinguishable syndromes in various species including man.

Susceptibility of different species to rabies and rabies related viruses.

Type	Virus	Species (in continent)	Other susceptible species
Genotype 1	Classical rabies virus	Carnivores, bats (in America)	All mammals
Genotype 2	Lagosbat virus	Frugivorous and insectivorous bats (in Africa)	Cat, dog, experimentally in monkey and mouse
Genotype 3	Mokola virus	Shrews and insectivorous rodents (in Africa)	Man
Genotype 4	Duvenhage virus	Insectivorous bats (in South Africa)	Man
Genotype 5	European bat lyssavirus 1	Insectivorous bats (*Eptesicus serotinus*) (In Europe)	Man, experimentally in mouse, cat and fox
Genotype 6	European bat lyssavirus 2	Insectivorous bats (*Eptesicus serotinus*) (In Europe)	Man
Genotype 7	Australian bat lyssa virus	Frugivorous and insectivorous bats (in Australia)	Man, experimentally in mouse and cat

The existence of a number of genotypes may have important implication in the vaccine production. The virus again has been grouped into street rabies virus and fixed rabies virus. The street virus is derived from one that exists in nature in naturally occurring cases and the fixed virus denotes to strains of virus that has been adapted by serial intracranial passage in rabbit in the laboratory. Fixed virus strains are used in the vaccine production. Fixed rabies virus causes paralytic disease with a relatively short incubation period following intracerebral inoculation and there is absence of Negri bodies and absence of virus in saliva and salivary glands.

Difference between street and fixed rabies viruses

Street rabies virus	Fixed rabies virus
Incubation period is long and variable.	Incubation period is short and fixed.
Rabbits die in 14 to 20 days following I/C inoculation of virus.	Rabbits die in 7 days following I/C inoculation of virus.
Negri bodies are present.	Negri bodies are not generally present.
Salivary glands are affected.	Salivary glands are not affected.

Inactivating agents : Lyssavirus is readily inactivated by heat, UV light, lipid solvent, formalin and other detergents e.g. Potassium permanganate, phenol, alkali and bichloride of mercury. Sunlight and moderate heat destroy the virus. The virus can be preserved in 50% glycerol and can survive in tissue culture at 37°C for a week.

Susceptible hosts : All warm blooded animals, with the possible exception of opossums, are susceptible and there is no difference in susceptibility in relation to age of the animals. Variation in susceptibility in different species is noticeable. Foxes, cotton rats and coyotes are extremely susceptible, cattle, rabbit and cats are highly susceptible and dogs, sheep and goats are moderately susceptible . Cattle and equidae may be considered as dead end hosts. The rabies virus is maintained by two different but interrelated cycle – urban cycle where disease transmission takes place through dogs and sylvatic cycle where the disease is transmitted through wildlife. Laboratory animals like swiss albino mice, guinea pigs and rabbits can experimentally be made susceptible by subdural, I/V, I/C and S/C inoculation. Rabies has been shown to affect blood, insect and fruit eating bats. The disease has been reported in 30 of 39 bat species resident in North America. In Latin America, virus transmitted by vampire bats is responsible for annual deaths of hundreds of thousands of cattle. Numerous human deaths are also attributed to vampire bats.

Mode of transmission : Transmission of rabies under natural conditions is commonly by bite of rabid animals usually carnivorous animals. The 90% of human cases occur due to the bite of rabid dog. In India, besides the problem in domestic animals like dog, cattle, cat etc, a limited survey reported the evidence of rabies in various species of rodents. Rabies infection also prevails in bandicoots, mongooses and rats. Death reports of human beings infected by other animals like dog, cat, fox, jackal, wolf, mongoose and rat bite were recorded in India.

Dogs are presumed to be the main transmitter (95%) in India. It is estimated that there is one dog in every 40 people and dog population is around 28 million. The infection is mostly transmitted by bite. A bite on the face has a contagion index of almost 100% whereas on the body or leg is about 25%.

The virus may also be transmitted through ingestion, inhalation and contamination of skin wounds by fresh saliva. Bats are important species in which symptomless carriers are known to occur. The virus multiplies in fatty tissues in bats without invasion of nervous symptom. Bats rarely show violent behaviour. The disease is most commonly noticed in late summer and autumn because wild animals move frequently for mating and in pursuit of food. Rabies virus can penetrate the mucous membrane of eyes, nose and mouth and thus aerosol infection is possible in a rabies laboratory by accident. Aerosol infection of man residing in cave or laboratory personnel has been reported.

Many clinically infected animals excrete virus in the saliva, particularly if infected with a relatively low dose of a homologous strain. The species difference exists in the duration of viral excretion before the onset of clinical signs. The period is short in cats (up to 24 hours), longer in dogs (up to 13 days) and longest in foxes (up to 29 days) following experimental infection. Apparently healthy carriers and excretors of rabies virus in saliva have been reported. The virus may be present in milk of affected animal but spread by this means is unlikely.

The infective virus travels centrifugally from peripheral nerves to the spinal cord and the brain. It then travels centripetally to the salivary glands prior to being in the brain.

The duration of incubation period depends on the following factors.

- Age of the animal : All age group of animals are equally susceptible if they are not immunized against rabies before.
- Distance of bite : The duration of incubation period depends on the site of the wound. In man, the virus can reach the brain from facial wound in 30 days, from the hand in 40 days and from the legs in 60 days.
- Virulence of virus : The severity of the disease would be increased with the enhanced virulence of the virus.
- Concentration of the virus : There is a correlation between the number of virus and the production of the disease.
- Degree of wound : The presence of hyaluronidase in the saliva has got the disease inducing effect. The saliva of the wild carnivores has a high content of hyaluronidase which is increased at the time of attack. The enzyme increases the permeability of the tissues and accelerates the virulence of the virus.

Pathogenesis : The usual route of rabies infection is transdermal inoculation of infected saliva. Airborne infection via mucous membrane was also documented almost exclusively to bat caves or laboratories where infectious aerosols are present. There is local replication of the virus in the epithelial cells or myocytes before the virus is taken up by the local nerve cells. Alternate pathway for spread of virus via blood or lymph in severe bite has also been suggested. The rabies virus glycoprotein attaches to the cells surface receptors which are expressed on various nerve, muscle cells, activated T cells and NK cells followed by uptake of the virus into the cell. The virus moves centripetally to the CNS via nervous pathways as the infection progresses.

After reaching the brain, virus invade ganglion cells and spread centrifugally to the peripheral nerves (facial, glossopharyngeal, trigeminal, olfactory) from the brain. In most of the cases, CNS lesions are typical of non-suppurative encephalitis with ganglioneuritis. The most significant lesions are generally in the pons, hypothalamus and cervical spinal cord. In later stages of the disease, the virus may also replicate in some non-neural tissues viz., the salivary glands, adrenals and cornea. However, in spite of spread along nerve routes, the brain remains the principal focus of infection and high concentrations of virus commonly occur in the cerebrum, hippocampus, medulla, thalamus and brainstem.

A characteristic feature of rabies is the long and variable incubation period during which virus is protected from the immune system within peripheral cells and nerves. The length of the incubation period depends on the site, dose and the virus strains involved. A short incubation period would be following a deep bite with large amount of virus near the head.

Epidemiology : Although most mammals are susceptible to rabies infection, classical rabies virus is particularly well adapted to small carnivores which are reservoir species throughout the world. In America, bats (Chiroptera) also transmit the disease. Spill over infection regularly occur in domestic animal and these animals increase the risk of human exposure. In developing countries, urban rabies in domestic dogs is often a serious public health problem whereas in developed countries, this disease is limited to wildlife population.

There are many strains of rabies virus that can be differentiated using MAbs or by sequencing genomic segments. Each strain is typically characteristic of a particular host species in which it is highly pathogenic. Infection is likely to result from a small infectious dose and the virus is excreted in high dose in saliva. Infection with a heterologous strain generally requires a higher infectious dose and sheds the virus in low titre in saliva. Thus canine rabies is readily maintained by a native population of dogs. However, virus adaptation to new host species continues to occur and leads to new epidemic cycles.

All the warm blooded animals are susceptible and there is no difference in susceptibility with relation to age of the animals. The susceptibility varies in different species. Animals like dog, fox, wolf, jackal, skunk, mongoose, cat, rat, squirrel and vampire bat are extremely susceptible in the tropical areas of the world. Cattle, goat and sheep are moderately susceptible. Cattle and Equidae used to remain as dead end hosts. Opossums (*Didelphis virginiana*) are resistant to rabies virus infection.

Clinical signs : Two types of clinical manifestations are noticed in dogs. They are furious form and dumb form. But this differentiation is not always perfect and one symptom may overlap with other.

(A) Furious form : In this form excitation is predominant changes and can be divided into stage of melanchology and stage of excitation.

Stage of melancholy : There is change of behaviour of the affected animal which does not obey its master. It often shows unusual violence and frenzy behaviour. The restrained dog may show the tendency to bite either nearby inanimate objects but set free dogs show the tendency to bite other animals and human beings which come across their ways till death. Rabid dog may move from one village to another in a circular manner (circling disease) thus spread the disease over wide areas.

Infected dog remains in unusual alert condition and respond very sharply to any stimulus. Dogs will snap or bite imaginary objects. Initially there is no deviation in appetite but later it becomes depraved (parvarted). There is an urge to chew or eat non-edible objects e.g. stone , bone, mud straw, grass or even their own faeces. The pupils get dilated and there is altered facial expression. Appetite is gradually suppressed but animal may lick water and attempt to drink water Due to paralysis of pharyngeal and laryngeal muscles the animal does not succeed to drink water. This period lasts for 1-3 days.

Stage of excitement : In this stage, dogs become aggressive due to increased excitability and irritability. Initially the animal will hide in dark place due to photophobia and will have the urge to bite. There is change in the bark which is very characteristic and due to paralysis of the vocal cord. There is champing of jaws and dribbling of saliva. The affected dogs will wander aimlessly and bite animals and persons who will come across its way. The affected animals will gradually show signs of emaciation, exhaustion and dejection. There will be in coordination and muscle tremors. Animals may lick their genitalia and bitch may show the signs of heat. At the end, the lower jaw will hang, tongue will protrude and head will drop down. There will be development of dyspnoea, ascending paralysis, coma and death. The episode may last as long as 10 days.

(B) Dumb form : It is also known as paralytic form. In this form there is paralysis of the lower jaw, tongue, larynx and hind quarters. The dogs can not bite, saliva remains infective and a peculiar voice is produced known as howl. There is hanging of jaws due to paralysis of jaw muscles. The dog used to seek solitude and appear sluggish and morosed. In the terminal stage of the disease dogs show progressive weakness and paralysis which cause them to stagger. There is coma and finally death. The episode lasts for 1-7 days.

Clinical signs in horse : The clinical signs of rabies in horse is similar to that of tetanus. Weakness or lameness is the initial sign. Horse may show furious form and become virulent and uncontrollable. The horse may fall on the ground, roll on the ground and chew foreign objects. There is drooling of saliva and convulsion. Horses may kick viciously and remain very destructive. Both mares and stallions may show transient period of sexual excitement. The horses refuses to eat its food and show dysphagia. It may eat inanimate objects. There is acceleration of pulse and respiratory rate and the whole episode lasts for 2-4 days.

Clinical signs in cattle and buffaloes : They show loss of appetite and sudden fall in milk yield. There is trembling, incoordination, paralysis of deglutition muscle with excessive salivation and grinding of teeth. There is difficulty in drinking of water simulating choke. Due to paralysis of vocal cord cattle will bellow incessantly in a low pitched voice. There is increased sexual excitement in both cow and bull.

Clinical signs in sheep and goat : Clinical signs are more or less similar to cattle and buffalo. There is increased sexual excitement, starring eyes, twitching of lips, salivation, aggression and continuous bleating. The course of the disease lasts for 2-6 days.

Clinical signs in pigs : Pig may become furious and attempt to bite inanimate objects. The signs are characterized by stoppage of food, violent movement, attempts of biting and death after a period of 4 days from the onset of signs.

Lesions : The lesions in rabies are limited to the central nervous system. The only macroscopical changes noticed may be hyperemia and oedema of the meninges with a few petechiae. Microscopically, non-suppurative encephalitis and perivascular cuffing of lymphocytes and plasma cells are noticed. The satellite cells proliferate around the ganglion cells to form small nodules – the Babes nodules which is first noticed in gasserian ganglion than in other parts. There is degeneration of ganglion cells and neuronophagia in hippocampus and the brain stem. Ganglioneuritis in perivascular ganglia is constantly found in rabies. These are swollen and red in colour and infiltrated with lymphocytes and degeneration and neuronophagia of ganglion cells. Besides, there is acute catarrh of the mucosa of the respiratory and digestive tracts, fullness of gall bladder, hyperemia of kidneys, spleen, liver and salivary glands. Negri bodies, acidophilic inclusion bodies contain basophilic granules found in the cytoplasm of the neurones are aggregates of the virus. They are round and have a halo round them. They are 1-27 μ in diameter and 1-20 bodies. They are also found in the dendrites of hippocampus. On the other hand, they are more numerous in the Purkinje's cells of the cerebellum.

Diagnosis : Laboratory diagnosis of rabies plays a pivotal role in the better management of both the biting and exposed animals and to control the epizootic.

1. On the basis of history and clinical signs.
2. A suspected dog must be kept isolated for at least 10 days. If rabid, it will die within that time.
3. Make impression smears of hippocampus and stain by Seller's stain or modified Mann's method and look for Negri bodies. Absence of Negri bodies in the impression smears does not exclude the possibility that the animal is non-rabid. Negri bodies may not be seen in positive cases.
4. Mouse inoculation test – 5% suspension of brain (hippocampus), salivary glands, saliva are to be made and inoculated I/C into 6 or more white mice (2-3 weeks old) with a volume of 0.03 ml. On 7 th day mice show symptoms. They are to be sacrificed and following test are to be done.

(a) Presence of Negri bodies – they appear on 5-6 day, but 10% case may not show Negri bodies.

(b) Search for infectivity – Infected mice brain suspension is to be inoculated into rabbit's brain for confirmation.

5. Complement fixation test : This test is carried out with brain tissues containing virus antigen with known antirabic serum.

6. Fluorescent antibody technique (FAT) : This test can be employed to detect the presence of rabies antigen in corneal smears, brain smears and smears from saliva or salivary glands. But the most suitable material for this test is brain. This test is considered superior in accuracy and comparative efficiency.

7. Immunoperoxidase test (IPT) : This test has been found to be better over FAT since this method does not require special kind of microscope and it can be kept for a long time. The impression smears can be prepared from brains.

8. Enzyme linked immunosorbent assay (ELISA) : With the advancement of the technology, hybridoma technique provides the monoclonal antibodies (MAbs), capable of detecting individual components of rabies virus, may replace the less selective polyclonal antibody in FAT. Enzyme has replaced the position of fluorescent dye in conjugate in immunoperoxidase test which is little less sensitive but it has the advantage of requiring only visible light instead of 'UV' sources and special optics. This immunoenzymatic system has been further developed into an ELISA type test, designated Rapid Rabies Enzyme Immuno-Diagnosis (RREID) in which both microscopy and fluorescence are unnecessary. In RREID, the ELISA plate is coated with the IgG raised against ribo-nucleoprotein (RNP) of Pasteur strain of rabies virus followed by the addition of homogenized suspected material same IgG conjugated with Horse Radish Peroxidase (HRPO) and finally substrate (OPD) solution. The optical density (OD) value was taken at 492 nm in an ELISA reader and compared with the OD values of known positive and negative samples. Another modification of the RREID is RREID-biotin, where IgG against RNP is conjugated with biotin instead of HRPO followed by addition of streptavidin-HRPO conjugate and substrate solution. The RREID-biotin is more sensitive than RREID test. Still another modification of RREID is RREID-lyssa where a mixture of IgG anti PV (Pasteur virus), EBL (European bat lyssavirus) and Mok-RNP (Mokola-ribonucleoprotein) is used to coat the ELISA plate. The rest of the procedure is similar to RREID except a mixture of same IgG anti RNP conjugated with HRPO. The prime purpose of this is to diagnose rabies along with the rabies related viruses which are becoming a great concern.

9. Molecular biological techniques : Further advances in the diagnosis of rabies has moved into the molecular arena, and dot hybridization was used to detect specific rabies RNA in brain material either from experimentally infected mice or submitted for routine diagnosis by using the complementary nucleic acid labeled with radio-isotope or non-radio-isotope markers. More recently, a polymerase amplification technique of viral nucleic acid has been reported as an alternative method for obtaining quick and accurate results in the diagnosis and epidemiological studies of rabies.

Differential Diagnosis

The diagnosis of rabies is important because of zoonotic importance and possible transmission of the virus to humans. Nervous signs may or may not be evident in the affected animals, so it also becomes difficult at times if they are affected by other affections and showing same neurological signs. Different species of animals can be suspected for possibility of rabies and can be differentially diagnosed from other diseases as: Listeriosis which is mainly manifested by facial nerve paralysis and circling movement. Enterotoxemia occurs only in lambs on high carbohydrate diets. Lactation tetany occurs in lactating cattle and is characterized by hyperaesthesia, tremors, convulsions, recumbency and death. Vitamin A deficiency occurs in young cattle and characterized by ocular blindness, tremors and convulsions. Acute and sub acute lead poisoning leads to convulsions, champing of jaw, grinding of teeth, stupor, blindness, frothy saliva and twitching of eyelids and ears. Blindness and convulsions and twitching of facial muscles do not occur in rabies. Bellowing, yawning, attacking and walking occurs in case of rabid cattle. Rabies should be differentiated from pseudorabies, African swine fever, erysipelas as these are also characterized by nervous signs and meningitis in case of pigs. In case of horses rabies should be differentiated from viral encephalomyelitis, Japanese Encephalitis, Borna, botulism and tetanus.

Preservation and dispatch of brain and salivary glands

Both the brain and the salivary glands can be sent to the laboratory through messenger or mail. Brain and salivary glands are packed in a glass or unbreakable plastic container containing 50% phosphate buffered saline and placed on ice in a ice-cool container for virological examination and diagnosis of the sample. For histopathological studies, part of the brain and salivary glands are to be kept in glass or plastic container containing 10% formol saline.

Treatment : There is no specific treatment for clinical rabies. Symptomatic treatments may be rendered with sedative and narcotic drugs. However, in the recent past, a large number of antiviral drugs have been tested against rabies virus. Many of them have the good chemotherapeutic index and great potential for use in treating rabid cases. But these are still confined to laboratory animals.

Vinkristin (Richter, Hungary) a suppressor of cellular immunity protected the mice if given a short time before or after wild rabies virus inoculation. IUDR (5-iodo 2 deoxy uridine) a nucleoside analogue afforded protection when given I/P in mice against challenge by wild rodent street virus. Scopolamide hydrobromide (Sigma, USA) a potent anticholinergic agent has been found effective against challenge rabies virus in mice. DPHA (9(s)2-3 dihydroxypropyl adenine) also protected the mice after oral administration against the challenge rabies virus. Interferon has a great potential in controlling rabies virus infection. Poly I or Poly C alone is not able to confer protection against rabies virus but Poly I:C which is a stable secondary structure and potent IFN inducer gives protection against rabies.

Vaccines : Antirabies vaccines employing a number of classical rabies virus strains and produced from sheep brain tissue are still used to vaccinate both human beings and animals in India. But there is always a perceived risk of anaphylactic shocks in vaccines due to the presence of myelin protein in the adult brain tissue. Subsequently mouse and rat brain derived vaccines having considerably low risk of anaphylactic shock have been available in the market. Later, anti-rabies vaccines of cell culture origin [Vero, BHK21, chicken embryo fibroblast (CEF), human diploid cell strain (HDCS)] replaced the conventional vaccines with side effects. Vaccines of cell culture origin are highly potent and efficacious and can be employed safely both in human beings and animals. Among all the vaccines, HDCS is receiving most attention. Flury's strains live attenuated vaccine (LEP) is used only in dogs whereas HEP is used to vaccinate other animals except dogs. The use of the new generation vaccines has enabled most developed countries to control the disease in domestic animal hosts and thus prevent the infection of human beings. However, the success of the vaccination campaign in developing countries depends on vaccine cost, the need for an effective cold chain and access to high proportion of the domestic dog populations.

With the implementation of appropriate vaccination programmes in domestic animals and human beings, rabies in the developed countries is largely a disease of wildlife population. European countries successfully controlled rabies in foxes by using live attenuated or recombinant oral vaccines. Similar projects targeting a variety of host species are underway in North America and elsewhere. The live vaccines are required to induce immunity after oral administration. A live recombinant vaccine in which the rabies glycoprotein gene was inserted into the genome of vaccinia virus has also been used successfully for oral vaccination of wildlife. Both live attenuated and live recombinant vaccines should be tested for any residual pathogenicity or genetic instability before being launched for large scale immunization. However, there is least possibility of rabies outbreak following use of live recombinant vaccine as it contains only a small part of rabies virus genome. Lastly, any vaccine should be thoroughly tested for safety, potency and innocuity before its use in target animals.

Pre and Post exposure immunization in animals : Although a number of new generation vaccines are available in the market, BPL inactivated brain tissue rabies vaccines (5%) are still being used to control the rabies in animals both in pre-exposure and post-exposure cases. The details of which has been given in the table.

Species of animals	**Dosage if the animal has never been immunized against rabies**	**Dosage if the animal has been immunized previously against rabies**
Animals weighing under 15 kg, e.g. dog, pup, cat, monkey etc.	2 ml daily for 14 days	2 ml daily for 7 days
Animals weighing 15-100 kg, e.g. dog, cat, sheep, goat, deer etc.	5 ml daily for 14 days	5 ml daily for 7 days
Animals weighing 100-800 kg, buffalo, bullock, cow, horse etc.	15 ml daily for 14 days	15 ml daily for 7 days
Animals weighing more than 800 kg, i.e. Camel, elephant etc.	30 ml daily for 14 days	30 ml daily for 7 days

Immunity : Rabies virus is highly neurotropic and remain largely protected from the cells of the immune system. Natural infection is characterized by little inflammatory response and the suppression of cell mediated immunity. The development of neutralizing antibodies is not an early feature of natural infection. Neither antibody nor virus is readily detected before the onset of clinical signs.

Immunization with an inactivated or attenuated virus and subsequently challenge is manifested by marked cell mediated immunity promoting cytotoxic lysis of infected cells, interferon production and marked antibody response. The attenuated rabies virus strains used in oral vaccination programmes induce abortive infection of the CNS with all the components of the immune system contributing to clearance of the virus. The anti-G antibody plays a pivotal role in the protection against rabies following challenge. Anti-nucleoprotein antibodies are also demonstrated following vaccination but their role is uncertain as it does not neutralize the virus.

The immune response to rabies vaccination following infection in native subjects is complex. The most important aspect of post-exposure treatment is the elimination of the virus before its uptake into nerve tissue. Thorough washing with soap or detergent immediately after bite is of extremely important as it neutralizes the virus. Neutralization of virus in-situ is very valuable and may be achieved by prompt administration of antibody together with vaccination. Following infection in man, the combination of human or equine rabies immunoglobulin and a potent and efficacious vaccine is nearly 100% effective in preventing the development of rabies when correctly and promptly administered. The result of post-exposure vaccination is variable both within and between species. If not administered promptly, it may be unsuccessful and result in either an accelerated or protracted clinical course. However, neutralizing antibody is of key importance and its use is never contraindicated.

Control : Following measures are to be adopted to control the disease. In India it has never been successful due to intermittent and erratic application of control strategies.

- Trained and skilled personnel are to be employed to study the know-how of the disease.
- Adequate transport facilities are to be provided to dispatch the materials for prompt and accurate diagnosis and to make available the requisite vaccine to control the outbreak.
- Administrative support should be there for disease investigation and control.
- There should be co-operation between veterinary and medical doctors to control the disease as it is a dreadly zoonotic disease.
- Research work should also be carried out to study the etiopathogenesis, aberrant course of the disease and to evolve the suitable vaccine.
- People's awareness should be increased through mass media, group discussion, seminar, symposium, leaflet and pamphlet.
- Strict measures are to be adopted to kill the street dogs.
- Systematic and exhaustive survey has to be undertaken to locate the problem.
- At least 70% of dog population should be vaccinated with L.E.P. vaccine in that immunity lasts for 3 years. Cats and cattle should be vaccinated with nervous tissue vaccine or HEP with annual vaccination.
- It should be made mandatory to vaccinate all the pet dogs against rabies through municipality and other statutory bodies.
- All the wild animals susceptible to rabies should be vaccinated with bait vaccine or other suitable vaccine.
- New generation cell culture based vaccines which are superior to conventional vaccines in inducing protective immunity and without side effects are to be used to immunize man and animals.

Further Reading

Amengual, B., Whitby, J.E., King, A., Cobo, S., and Bourhy, H. (1997). Evolution of European bat lyssavirus. *J. Gen. Virol.* 78: 2319-2328.

Artois, M., Cliquet, F., Barrat, J. and Schumacher, C.L. (1997). Effectiveness of SAG1 oral vaccine for the long-term protection of red foxes (*Vulpes vulpes*) against rabies. *Vet. Rec.* 140: 57–59.

Badrane, H., Bahloul, C., Perrin, P. and Tordo, N. (2001). Evidence of two Lyssavirus phylogroups with distinct pathogenicity and immunogenicity. *J. Virol.* 75: 3268-3276.

Bahloul, C., Taieb, D., Diouani, MF., Ahmed, S.B., Chtourou, Y. and B'chir, B.I. (2006). Field trials of a very potent rabies DNA vaccine which induced long lasting virus neutralizing antibodies and protection in dogs in experimental conditions. *Vaccine.* 24(8): 1063–1072.

Blanton, J.D., Hanlon, C.A. and Rupprecht, C.E. (2007). Rabies surveillance in the United States during 2006. *J. Amer. Vet. Med. Assoc.* 231(4): 540–56.

Black, E.M., McElhinney, L.M., Lowings, J.P., Smith, J., Johnstone, P. and Heaton, P.R. (2000). Molecular methods to distinguish between classical rabies and the rabies related European bat lyssaviruses. *J. Virol. Meth.* 87(12): 123-131.

Bourhy, H., Kissi, B. and Tordo, N. (1993). Molecular diversity of the *Lyssavirus* genus. *Virology.* 194: 70-81.

Briggs, D.J., Banzhoff, A. and Nicolay, U. (2000). Antibody response of patients after post-exposure rabies vaccination with small intradermal doses of puriûed chick embryo cell vaccine or puriûed vero cell rabies vaccine. *Bull. W.H. O.* 78(5): 693–698.

Burton, E.C., Burnsm, D.K., Opatowsky, M.J., El-Feky, W.H., Fischbach, B., Melton, L., Sanchez, E., Randall,H. and Chang, J. (2005). Rabies encephalomyelitis: clinical, neuro-radiological and pathological findings in 4 transplant recipients. *Arch. Neurol.* 62(6): 873–882.

Chaudhuri, S. (2005). Rabies prevention and dog population management. India's official dog control policy in context of WHO guidelines. *Ecollage.* 2005.

Chulasugandha, P., Khawplod, P., Havanond, P. and Wilde, H. (2006). Cost comparison of rabies pre-exposure vaccination with post-exposure treatment in Thai children. *Vaccine.* 24(9): 1478-1482.

Cleaveland, S. (1998). Epidemiology and control of rabies – The growing problem of rabies in Africa. *Transactions of the Royal Society of Tropical Medicine and Hygiene.* 92: 131–134.

Cliquet, F. and Picard-Meyer, E. (2004). Rabies and rabies-related viruses: a modern perspective on an ancient disease. *Revue Sci. Tech. (OIE).* 23(2): 625-642.

Cliquet, F., Gurbuxami, J.P., Pradhan, H.K., Pattnaik, B., Patil, S.S. and Regnault, A. (2007). Safety and efficacy of the oral rabies vaccine SAG2 in Indian stray dogs. *Vaccine.* 25: 3409–18.

Davis, P.L., Holmes, E.C., Larrous, F., Vander-Poel, W.H.M., Tjornehoj, K., Alonso, W.J. and Bourhy, H. (2005). Phylogeography, Population Dynamics and Molecular Evolution of European Bat Lyssaviruses. *J. Virol.* 79(16): 10487-10497.

Dietzschold, B., Faber, M. and Schnell, M.J. (2003). New approaches to the prevention and eradication of rabies. *Expert Review Vaccines.* 2: 399–406.

Dietzschold, B. and Schnell, M.J. (2002). New approaches to the development of live attenuated rabies vaccines. *Hybrid Hybridomics* 21: 129–134.

Dreesen, D.W. and Hanlon, C.A. (1998). Current recommendations for the prophylaxis and treatment of rabies. *Drugs.* 56: 801–809.

Dressen, D.W. (1997). A global review of rabies vaccines for human use. *Vaccine* 15: S2–6.

Fooks, A.R., Brookes, S.M., Johnson, N., Mc Elhinney, L.M. and Hutson, A.M. (2003). European bat lyssaviruses: an emerging zoonosis. *Epid. Infect.* 131: 1029-1039.

Hanlon, C.A., Kuzmin, I., Blanton, J., Manangan, J., Murphy, S.M. and Rupprecht, C.E. (2003). Efûcacy of biologics against newly described lyssaviruses. In: Proceedings of 14th International conference on Rabies in the Americas, pp. 55–56.

Hanlon, C.A., Kuzminm I.V., Blanton, J.D., Weldon, W.C., Manangan, J.S. and Rupprecht, C.E. (2005). Efficacy of rabies biologics against new lyssaviruses from Eurasia. *Virus Research.* 111: 44-54.

Hanlon, C.A., Niezgoda, M. and Rupprecht, C.E. (2002).Post-exposure prophylaxis for prevention of rabies in dogs. *Amer. J. Vet. Res.* 63: 1096–100.

Haupt, W. (1999). Rabies-risk of exposure and current trends in prevention of human cases. *Vaccine.* 17(13-14): 1742-1749.

Hoque, M., Islam, T., Das, S.C., Jabeen, N. and Islam, T. (2006). An overview of rabies in man and animals. *Intas Polivet.* **7:** 388–98.

Hu, R.L., Zhang, S.F., Fooks, A.R., Yuan, H., Liu, Y. and Li, H. (2006). Prevention of rabies virus infection in dogs by a recombinant canine adenovirus type-2 encoding the rabies virus glycoprotein. *Microbes and Infection.* 8: 1090-7.

Hu, R., Liu, Y., Zhang, S., Zhang, F. and Fooks, A.R. (2007).Experimental immunization of cats with a recombinant rabies-canine adenovirus vaccine elicits a long-lasting neutralizing antibody response against rabies. *Vaccine* 25(29): 5301–7.

Jaiiaroensup, W., Lang, J. and Thipkong, P. (1998). Safety and effieacy of purified vero cell rabies vaccine given intramuscularly and intradermally (results of a prospective randomized trial). *Vaccine* 16(16): 1559–62.

Jakel, V., Cussler, K., Konig, M. and Thiel, H.J. (2007). Factors inûuencing the antibody response to rabies vaccination. In: Joint OIE/WHO/EU International Conference: "Towards the Elimination of Rabies in Eurasia". Advances in Technologies, Diagnosis and Vaccines, Paris, May, pp. 27–30.

Jayakumar, R., Ramadass, P. and Raghavan, N. (1989). Studies on immune response and protective capacity of rabies vaccine in Indian dogs. *Revue Sci. Tech. (OIE)* 8: 199–208.

John, T.J. (1997). An ethical dilemma in rabies immunisation. *Vaccine.* 15: S12-15.

Kallel, H., Jouini, A., Majoul, S. and Rourou, S. (2002). Evaluation of various serum and animal protein free media for the production of a veterinary rabies vaccine in BHK-21 cells. *J. Biotech.* 95: 195-204.

Kamoltham, T., Khawplod, P. and Wilde, H. (2002). Rabies intradermal post-exposure vaccination of humans using reconstituted and stored vaccine. *Vaccine.* 20: 3272–6.

Kamoltham, T., Singhsa, J., Promsaranee, U., Sonthon, P., Mathean, P. and Thinyounyong, W. (2003). Elimination of human rabies in a canine endemic province in Thailand: five-year programme. *Bull. W.H.O.* 81(5): 375–81.

Kamoltham, T., Thinyounyong, W., Phongchamnaphai, P., Phraisuwan, P., Khawplod, P. and Banzhoff, A. (2007). Pre-exposure rabies vaccination using puriûed chick embryo cell rabies vaccine intradermally is immunogenic and safe. *J. Pediatrics* 151(2): 173–7.

Katie, H., Jonathan, D., John, B., Gideon, B., Ali, Y.H. and Andy, D. (2007). Synchronous cycles of domestic dog rabies in sub-Saharan Africa and the impact of control efforts. *PNAS.* 104(18): 7717-7722.

Khawplod, P., Wilde, H., Tantawichien, T., Limusanno, S., Tantawichien, T. and Mitmoonpitak, C. (2002). Potency, sterility and immunogenicity of rabies tissue culture vaccine after reconstitution and refrigerated storage for 1 week. *Vaccine.* 20: 2240–2.

Kieny, M.P., Lathe, R., Drillien, R., Spehner, D., Skory, S. and Schmitt, D. (1990). Expression of rabies virus glycoprotein from a recombinant vaccinia virus. *Nature.* 312: 163-6.

Kihm, U., Flamand, A., Pastoret, P.P. and Peterhans, E. (1992). Round table on epidemiology and control of fox rabies. *Vet. Microbiol.* 33(1-4): 297-301.

Knobel, D.L., Cleaveland, S., Coleman, P.G., Fevre, E.M., Meltzer, M.I., Miranda, M.E., Shaw, A., Zinsstag, J. and Meslin, F.X. (2005). Reevaluating the burden of rabies in Africa and Asia. *Bull. W.H.O.* 83: 360-368.

Lambot, M., Blasco, E., Barrat, J., Cliquet, F., Brochier, B., Renders, C., Krafft, N., Bailly, J., Munier, M., Aubert, M.F.A. and Pastoret, P.P. (2001). Humoral and cell-mediated immune responses of foxes (*Vulpes vulpes*) after experimental primary and secondary oral vaccination using SAG 2 and V-RG vaccines. *Vaccine.* 19: 1827–1835

Lang, J. and Wood, S.C. (2000). Development of orphan vaccine - an industry perspective. *Emer. Infect. Dis.* 5 : 749-756.

Lodmell, D.L., Smith, J.S., Esposito, J.J. and Ewalt, L.C. (1995). Cross-protection of mice against a global spectrum of rabies virus variants. *J. Virol.* **69:** 4957–62.

Lodmell, D.L., Ray, N.B. and Ewalt, L.C. (1998). Gene gun particle-mediated vaccination with plasmid DNA confers protective immunity against rabies virus infection. *Vaccine.* 16(2): 115–8.

Lodmell, D.L. and Ewalt, L.C. (2000). Rabies vaccination: comparison of neutralizing antibody responses after priming and boosting with different combinations of DNA, inactivated virus, or recombinant vaccinia virus vaccines. *Vaccine.* 18(22): 2394–8.

Lodmell, D.L. and Ewalt, L.C. (2004). Rabies cell culture vaccines reconstituted and stored at 4 °e%C for 1 year prior to use protect mice against rabies virus. *Vaccine*. 22: 3237–3239.

Madhusudana, S.N., Anand, N.P. and Shamsundar, R. (2002). Economical multi site intradermal regimen with purified chick embryo cell vaccine (Rabipur) prevents rabies in people bitten by confirmed rabid animals. *Int. J. Infectious Dis.* 6: 210–4.

Madhusudana, S.N., Sanjay, T.V., Mahendra, B.J., Sudarshan, M.K., Narayana, D.H. and Giri, A. (2006). Comparison of safety and immunogenicity of purified chick embryo cell rabies vaccine (PCECV) and purified vero cell rabies vaccine (PVRV) using the Thai Red Cross intradermal regimen at a dose of 0.1ml. *Vaccine.* 2(5): 200–4.

Mansûeld, K.L., Burr, P.D., Snodgrass, D.R., Sayers, R. and Fooks, A.R. (2004). Factors affecting the serological response of dogs and cats to rabies vaccination. *Vet. Rec.* 154(14): 423–426.

Masson, E., Bruyere-Masson, V., Vuillaume, P., Lemoyne, S. and Aubert, M. (1999). Rabies oral vaccination of foxes during the summer with the VRG vaccine bait. *Vet. Res.* 30(6): 595–605.

Messenger, S.L., Rupprecht, C.E. and Smith, J.S. (2003). Bats, emerging virus infections, and the rabies paradigm. In Bat ecology (T.H. Kunz & M.B. Fenton, eds). University of Chicago Press, Chicago, 622-667.

Ming, L., Todd, J.G., Xin, Z., Jun, T. and Shihong, Q. (2007). Conserved characteristics of the rhabdovirus nucleoprotein. *Virus Research.* 129(2): 246-251.

Moore, S.M., Ricke, T.A., Davis, R.D. and Briggs, D.J. (2005). The influence of homologous versus heterologous challenge virus strains on the serological test results of rabies neutralization assays. *Biologicals*. 33: 269-276.

Morimoto, K., McGettigan, J.P., Foley, H.D., Hooper, D.C., Dietzschold, B. and Schnell, M.J. (2001). Genetic engineering of live rabies vaccines. *Vaccine.* 19: 3543–3551.

Nagarajan, T., Mohanasubramanian, B., Seshagiri, E.V., Nagendrakumar, S.B., Saseendranath, M.R., Satyanarayana, M.L., Thiagarajan, D., Rangarajan, P.N. and Srinivasan, V.A. (2006). Molecular epidemiology of rabies virus isolates in India. *J. Clin. Microbiol.* 44(9): 3218–3224.

Nandi, S. (2002). Epidemiology of wildlife rabies. *Indian Farming.* 51 : 12 : 26-28.

Nandi, S. (2002). Rabies – a new look to an old disease. *Indian Farming.* 52 :2 : 34-37.

Nandi, S. (2002). Recent advances in immunoprophylaxis against rabies. *Indian Farming.* 52 : 5 : 27-30.

Nandi, S. (2006). Guidelines for management of post-exposure rabies cases. *Indian Farming.* 55 : 10 : 28-30.

Nandi, S., Saha, S.K., Katole, S. and Samanta, M.K. (2008). Origin of Rabies virus vaccine strains. *Livestock Line.* 2: 3 : 15-18.

Nandi, S. (2008). Intradermal rabies immunization : effective and affordable pre and post exposure prophylaxis. *Indian Farming.* 58 : 10 : 24-27.

Nandi, S. and Yadav, J.S. (2010). Carrier state of rabies – a genuine problem. *Indian Farming.* 59 : 10 : 30-32.

Nandi, S., Audarya, S.D., Suresh, I. and Chauhan, R.S. (2006). Emergence of Rabies and Rabies related Viruses – a Real Challenge. 7th All India Conference of The Association of Public Health Veterinarians (APHV) and National Symposium on "Prospective Role of Veterinary Public Health in Integrated Rural Development" held at College of Veterinary Science and Animal Husbandry, O.U.A.T., Bhubaneswar, Orissa from Dec. 7-8, pp 83-89.

Nandi, S. (2008). Molecular basis of rabies virus virulence with special reference to wildlife. Global meet on Veterinary Public Health and Symposium on "New Horizons in Food Security with special reference to Veterinary Public Health and Hygiene – Evolving Strategies with Global Perspectives" and 8th Convention of APHV held at Lucknow from November 19-21, pp 196-204.

Nandi, S. and Kumar, M. (2010). Development in immunoprophylaxis against Rabies for animals and humans. *Avicenna Journal Medical Biotechnology.* 2 : 1 : 3-21.

Nandi, S. and Kumar, M. (2011). Global perspective of rabies and rabies related viruses : a comprehensive review. *Asian J. Anim. Vet. Adv.* 6 (2) : 101-116.

Nandi, S. and Chauhan, R.S. (2006). Rabies and Rabies Related Viruses - A Perspective. Lead paper presented in the International Symposium and 5th Annual Conference on "New Strategies for Prevention and Control of Emerging and Reemerging Zoonoses – An Integrated Veterinary and Medical Approach" held at Department of Veterinary Public Health, CSKHPAU, Palampur, H.P., India from October 12-14, 2006.

Nandi, S. (2010). Global perspective of rabies and rabies related viruses : a comprehensive review. Lead paper presented in National Congress on Canine Practice and 7th Annual Convention of ISACP on "Novel Approaches in Companion Animal Practice" held at Atria Hotel and Veterinary College, KVAFSU, Hebbal, Bangalore from 21-23th January, 2010. pp 113-126.

Nandi, S., Goel, A.C. and Pandey, K.D. (1990). Immunogenic response to partially purified rabies virus as measured by ELISA. *Indian J. Virol.* 6:1-2: 89-92.

Nandi, S. and Maiti, S.K. (1996). Twenty salient points about rabies. *Asian Livestock (FAO).* XXI :3: 35-36.

Nandi, S. and Maiti, S.K. (1995). When should your pets get vaccination against rabies. *Asian Livestock (FAO).* XX: 4: 46-48.

Nandi, S. and Tiwari, A.K. (1994). Rabies in bats. *Asian Livestock (FAO).* XIX :4: 47-48.

Nandi, S. and Tiwari, A.K. (1994). Chemotherapeutic agents against rabies. *Asian Livestock (FAO).* XIX :9: 105-107.

Nandi, S. and Maiti, S.K. (1994). Recent advances in the diagnosis of rabies. *Asian Livestock (FAO).* XIX :11: 150-152.

Nandi, S., Pandey, K.D and Goel, A.C. (1990). Partial purification of rabies virus from brain tissue by sonication and treatment with PEG and genetron. *Indian J. Comp. Microbiol. Immunol. Infect. Dis.* 11:1: 1-6.

OIE (World organisation for animal health) (2004). Rabies. In: OIE Manual of standards for diagnostic tests and vaccines, 5th ed. OIE, Paris, pp. 276–291.

Osorio, J.E., Tomlinson, C.C., Frank, R.S., Haanes, E.J., Rushlow, K. and Haynes, J.R. (1999). Immunization of dogs and cats with a DNA vaccine against rabies virus. *Vaccine.* 17(9–10): 1109–16.

Pastoret, P.P., Kappeler, A. and Aubert, M. (2004). European rabies control and its history. In: King AA, Fooks AR, Aubert M, Wandeler AI, editors. Historical perspective of rabies in Europe and the Mediterranean basin. Paris: OIE; p. 337–47.

Perrin, P., Jacob, Y., Aguilar-Setien, A., Loza-Rubio, E., Jallet, C., Desmezieres, E., Aubert, M., Cliquet, F. and Tordo, N. (2000). Immunization of dogs with a DNA vaccine induces protection against rabies virus. *Vaccine.* 18: 479–86.

Quiambao, B.P., Dimaano, E.M., Ambas, C., Davis, R., Banzhoff, A. and Malerzcyk, C. (2005). Reducing the cost of post-exposure rabies prophylaxis: *efficacy* of 0.1ml PCEC rabies vaccine administered intradermally using the Thai Red Cross post-exposure regimen in patients severely exposed to laboratory-confirmed rabid animals. *Vaccine.* 23(14): 1709–14.

Rupprecht, C.E. and Gibbons, R.V. (2004). Prophylaxis against Rabies. *New England J. Med.* 351(25): 2626 - 2635.

Schneider, M.C., Belotto, A., Ade, M.P., Hendrickx, S., Leanes, L.F., Rodrigues, M.J., Medina, G. and Correa, E. (2007). Current status of human rabies transmitted by dogs in Latin America. *Cad Saude Publica* 23(9): 2049-2063.

Shayam, C., Duggal, A.K., Kamble, U. and Agarwal, A.K. (2006). Post-exposure prophylaxis for rabies. *J. Indian Academy of Clin. Med.* 7: 39–46.

Singh, C.K. and Sandhu, B.S. (2007). Epidemiological investigation of rabies in Punjab. *Indian J. Anim. Sci.* 77: 653-658.

Slater, M.R. (2001). The role of veterinary epidemiology in the study of free-roaming dogs and cats. *Preventive Veterinary Medicine.* 48(4): 273-286.

Sudarshan, M.K. (2004). Assessing burden of rabies in India. WHO sponsored national multi-centric rabies survey. *Assoc. for Prev. Cont. Rabies India.* 6: 44-45.

Sudarshan, M.K., Madhusudana, S.N., Mahendra, B.J., Narayana, D.H.A., Giri, M.S.A., Popova, O. and Vakil, H.B. (2005). Evaluation of a new five-injection, two-site, intradermal schedule for purified chick embryo cell rabies vaccine: A randomized, open-label, active-controlled trial in healthy adult volunteers in India. *Current Therapy Research in Clinical Experiment* 66(4): 323-334.

Sudarshan, M.K., Madhusudana, S.N., Mahendra, B.J., Rao, N.S., Ashwath, N.D.H. and Abdul, R.S. (2007). Assessing the burden of human rabies in India: results of a national multi-center epidemiological survey. *Int. J. Infect. Dis.* 11: 29–35.

Sugiyamaa, M. and Ito, N. (2007). Control of rabies: Epidemiology of rabies in Asia and development of new-generation vaccines for rabies. *Comp. Immunol. Microbiol. Infect. Dis.* 30: 273–286.

Tuffereau, C., Leblois, H., Benejean, J., Coulon, P., Lafay, F. and Flamand, A. (1989). Arginine or lysine in position 333 of ERA and CVS glycoprotein is necessary for rabies virulence in adult mice. *Virology* 172: 206–12.

Vos. A., Neubert, A., Aylan, O., Schuster, P., Pommerening, E., Muller, T. and Chivatsi, D.C. (1999). An update on safety studies of SAD B19 rabies virus vaccine in target and non-target species. *Epid. Infect.* 123: 165–175.

Vos, A., Neubert, A., Pommerening, E., Muller, T., Dohner, L., Neubert, L. and Hughes, K. (2001). Immunogenicity of an E1-deleted recombinant human adenovirus against rabies by different routes of administration. *J. Gen. Virol.* 82: 2191–2197.

Wang, Y., Xiang, Z., Pasquiru, S., Ertl, H.C.J.(1998). Effect of passive immunization or maternally transferred immunity on the antibody response to a genetic vaccine to rabies virus. *J. Virol.* 72: 1790–6.

Wilde, H., Khawplod, P., Khamoltham, T., Hemachudha, T., Tepsumethanon, V., Lumlerdacha, B., Mitmoonpitak, C. and Sitprija, V. (2005). Rabies control in South and Southeast Asia. *Vaccine.* 23(17-18): 2284-2289.

Wilde, H. and Hemachudha, T. (2006). How far can the antigen content of tissue culture rabies vaccine be reduced safely? *Vaccine.* 24(10): 1489-1493.

Woldehiwet, Z. (2002). Rabies: recent developments. *Res. Vet. Sci.* 73: 17–25.

World Health Organisation (1996). Laboratory Techniques in Rabies, Fourth Edition, Meslin F.X., Kaplan M.M. & Koprowski H., eds. WHO, Geneva, Switzerland.

World Health Organization (WHO) (2001). Strategies for the control and elimination of rabies in Asia. Report of a WHO interregional consultation. Report of the workshop on rabies control in Asian countries, 17-21 July, Geneva. WHO, Geneva, 32 pp.

Wunderli, .PS., Dreesen, D.W., Miller, T.J. and Baer, G.M. (2003). Effect of heterogeneity of rabies virus strain and challenge route on efficacy of inactivated rabies vaccines in mice. *Amer. J. Vet. Res.* 64(4): 499–505.

❑❑❑

4

Peste Des Petits Ruminants (PPR)

Synnoyms : Pseudorinderpest, Goat plaque, Goat catarrhal fever

It is a severe rinderpest like disease of small ruminants viz., sheep, goat and wild ruminants characterized by pyrexia, catarrhal inflammation of ocular and nasal mucous membrane, erosive stomatitis, enteritis and pneumonia. The disease is also called goat plaque, kata, pseudorinderpest and stomatitis pneumo-enteritis complex. The current and standard name of the disease was chosen by the International Workshop of the disease in Ibadan, Nigeria, 1980.

Distribution : PPR first reported in 1942 in Ivory Coast by Gargadennec and Lalanne. For long time, PPR was confined to West Africa, but now it exists in East Africa, from sub-saharan Africa to Arabian Peninsula, the middle East, Bangladesh, Nepal, Pakistan and India. For the first time in India, Shaila *et al.,* (1989) isolated PPR virus from T.N. and confirmed it by cDNA probes. Subsequently, outbreaks in sheep and goat were reported from other parts of T.N., A.P., Karnataka, Maharashtra, Rajasthan, U.P., H.P. and W.B. during 1992-1995. It was earlier confined to Southern India and is now widely distributed in whole Indian subcontinent.

Etiology : The etiological agent of PPR is a virus under the genus *Morbillivirus* and family *Paramyxoviridae.* Other members of the same genus include canine distemper virus, RP virus and Measles virus. PPR viruses are pleomorphic in shape (spherical as well as filamentous forms occur) and 150-300 nm in diameter. Virions are enveloped, covered with large peplomers (8-20 nm in length), and contain a 'herring bone shaped' helically symmetrical nucleocapsid of 600-800 nm in length and 18 nm in diameter. The genome consists of a single linear molecule of negative sense, SS RNA of 15-16 kb in size. Morbillivirus contain 6 genes coding for structural proteins found in virions. The peplomers are composed of two proteins haemagglutinin (HA) and fusion protein (F). Both proteins play important role in the pathogenesis of all paramyxovirus infections. The HA protein elicits neutralizing antibodies that inhibit adsorption of virus to cellular receptors. The fusion protein is present on the newly formed virions in an inactive precursor form that is cleaved by a cellular protease. The cleavage of the fusion protein is essential for viral infectivity.

The PPR virus and RP virus are the two candidates within the same family and genus causing disease in small and large ruminants respectively but are not rigidly species specific. Both can infect large and small ruminants. In nature, these viruses maintain a separate and independent existence with a distinct epidemiology. Generally, PPR virus infects small ruminants and RP virus causes disease in large ruminants However, there have been reports of PPR virus causing subclinical infection in cattle without spreading the virus to in contact animals and RPV causing clinical and subclinical disease in small ruminants.

Susceptible hosts : PPR is a rinderpest like disease of sheep and goats. Clinical signs and pathological lesions are confusingly similar to those of RP. Both sheep and goats are susceptible to PPR but goats are more susceptible than sheep in field outbreaks. The young, adult and both the sexes of sheep and goats are susceptible. PPR virus does not attack cattle, buffaloes and pigs under natural conditions. Experimentally, cattle have been infected without clinical signs and resisted experimental challenge inoculation with virulent RP virus suggesting PPR virus conferring cross protection against RP virus in animals. Similarly, PPR virus infected goats transferred infection to contact pigs, but pig to pig transmission did not occur. PPR in wildlife has also been reported. The disease has also been reported in a variety of wild animals viz., dorcas gazelle (*Gazella dorcas species*) , dama gazelle (*Gazella dama*) nilgai (*Bosephalus tragocamelus*), Nubian ibex (*Capra ibex nubiana*), red deer (*Cervus elaphus*), Laristan sheep (*Ovis orientalis laristanica*), gemsbok (Oryx gazelle) etc.

Mode of transmission

- Natural infection occurs mainly through direct contact with infected sheep or goat.
- Secretions, excretions and faeces contain high concentration of virus and spread of the disease take place through inanimate objects contaminated with it like RP.
- There is no carrier state in animal but disease can be spread through animals with subclinical infection.
- The disease is also transmitted through ingestion of infected materials or inhalation.
- There is no insect vector which can transmit the disease but wild ruminants may play a role in the spreading of the disease.
- The disease has been introduced in many countries particularly Middle

East through importation of sick sheep, goat and their meat products from Africa.

- Most of the disease outbreaks occur in wet months when rainfall causes goats to hurdle together enhancing the air borne transmission. The virus survives for long time in nature if high relative humidity persists.

Pathogenesis : After entry into the body, the virus invades the retropharyngeal lymph node and both alimentary and respiratory tract mucosa are affected. Inflammation of alimentary tract mucosa causes enteritis and diarrhoea, dehydration and death in young animals. Pneumonia and respiratory distress are due to inflammation of respiratory tract mucosa. Young goat may die due to anoxic anoxia. The disease may be further complicated by secondary infections. Bacteria like *E. coli* and Pasteurella and protozoa like coccidia have been found to be associated with PPR to aggravate the condition. Animals may die due to severe pneumonia and death. Recovered animals may develop life long immunity.

Clinical signs : The clinical signs of acute PPR in goats and sheep is fever (39-41°C) after an incubation period of 6 days. There is profuse serous and nasal and ocular discharges which may turn from mucopurulent to purulent. Some may show signs of conjunctivitis. There is increased respiration rate (120/minutes) with extended head and mouth breathing. Signs of pneumonia become prominent and animal may die due to respiratory distress.

The lesions are found in alimentary tract mucosa. Necrotic lesions are evident in lip, buccal mucosa (stomatitis), gum (gingivitis), dental pad, palate and tongue accompanied with odematous lips. Diarrhoea is most commonly observed after 3-4 days and faeces contain mucous and blood. Due to diarrhea, emaciation and dehydration set in, temperature goes down, animals become exhausted and finally death occurs. Subacute form is mostly seen in sheep with signs of acute form in lower grade. A typical forms occur as abortion, nervous symptoms and vulvovaginitis.

Experimental PPR infection led to gradual decline in plasma volume, serum sodium and potassium values in goats. This was pronounced on day 10 when diarrhea was severe. There were no significant changes in chloride, bicarbonate, phosphate, urea, total protein and albumin in the disease. The virus has destructive effect on lymphocytes.

Lesions : These are mostly alike in the two diseases. The most prominent pathological lesions such as erosions in the lips, dental pad, tongue, soft and hard palate and cheeks, esophagus, pillars of the rumen, abomasums and intestine, conjunctivitis and gastroenteritis. There is pronounced necrosis of lymphocytes in lymph nodes, tonsil, Payer's patches and spleen. The distinguishing pathological features between RP and PPR is the frequent occurrence of primary broncho-interstitial pneumonia in the latter disease. This is due to the affinity of the virus to bronchial epithelial cells and alveolar macrophages which are infected and destroyed.

Histopathologically, there is degeneration of epithelial cells at the edge of erosions of the oral mucosa in experimentally infected sheep and goat. Lymph nodes showed depletion of lymphoid cells, infiltration of macrophage in the germinal centres and sinuses and pyknosis and karyorrhexis of lymphoid cells. Lymph nodes in the head regions were haemorrhagic, necrotic and depletion of lymphoid cells. Spleen exhibited extensive haemorrhages, necrosis and hemosiderin deposits. Interstitial pneumonia with occasional eosinophilic nuclear inclusion body in the pneumocytes. In the lungs , there are many I/ nuclear and I/cytoplasmic inclusions and alveolar giant cells. In the small intestine there are degenerated villi, in the cellular casts in the crypts and depletion of lymphoid cells in the Payer's patches and eosinophilic nuclear inclusions in the epithelial cells. Sections of the small and large intestine had ulcerated mucosa and submucosal haemorrhages.

Diagnosis : It is based on history, clinical signs and haematological observations and laboratory tests.

(a) Haematological examination : 1) Haemconcentration 2) Hyponatraemia 3) Hypocalaemia 4) Leucopenia 5) Hypokalemia.

An accurate diagnosis of PPR is quite impossible under field condition. The disease can be easily mistaken for RP, BT or FMD. However, a distinguishing feature is the presence of lameness in the last two diseases. Blue tongue is also characterized by muscle weakness, fatique and pain.

Laboratory diagnosis of the PPR is done either by serological test or recently developed non serological tests. Various techniques have been applied in the serological diagnosis of PPR in sheep and goats. These include AGPT, CIE, VNT, ELISA (indirect, competititon and immunocapture). Differential electrophoretic profile in the 'N' protein, nucleic acid hybridization using either radio-labelled or biotynated c-DNA probes and RT-PCR using P and F gene specific primers have been used for precise, correct and reliable diagnosis of PPR from RP. However, ELISA using MAbs against either 'N', 'H' or recombinant 'N' protein could differentiate PPR from RP. Immune electron microscopy using ferritin conjugated antibodies can differentiate PPR from RP but expensive and sophisticated instrument is necessary. Serum neutralization test using homologous and heterologus viruses and sera could differentiate PPR from RP but the test is time consuming, cumbersome and require viable viruses in the field sample.

Differential diagnosis : The disease should be differentiated from RP, BT, FMD, *E. coli*, coccidia and C.C.P.P. It is virtually impossible to differentiate it from RP based mainly on clinical signs. Confirmatory diagnosis can be achieved by carrying out serological test.

Treatment : There is no specific treatment against this disease. Symptomatic treatment may be provided for diarrhoea and respiratory problem. Fluid therapy may be given to restore the fluid loss and antibiotics may be suggested to check the bacterial infection. Hyper immune RP and PPR serum may be administered in affected animals. Specific antibiotic, intestinal sedative and electrolyte therapy were used for the treatment of pneumonia, diarrhoea and the restoration of the body ionic balance. There is no specific treatment for the labial scabs. Lemon fruit scrubbing, iodine-aureomycin spray and tincture of iodine have been proved effective and within 6 days labial scabs were cleared completely. The quick clearance of the labial scabs enhances early return of the animal to normal feeding ability and good nursing and warm draught free environment is a prerequisite for the proper management and early recovery of clinical cases.

Control : PPR is endemic in India. There are lot of outbreaks reported in the country throughout the year. Legislative control of animal movement and slaughter of affected animals is not feasible. The only effective way to control the disease is preventive vaccination. Besides, strict sanitation and hygienic measures are to be adopted in flock. The new animal from disease prone area should not be introduced in a flock. Sick animals purchased from market should not be allowed to mingled with healthy animals without keeping in quarantine for a finite period.

Vaccines : Tissue culture rinderpest vaccine has been proved to be effective against PPR as it confers satisfactory level of cross immunity. Vaccine should be administered at 3-4 months of age when there is little or no maternal antibodies. The vaccine can be used in an actual outbreak to protect the animals after keeping them segregated from the infected ones for a week or two because there is a risk that some animals already may be incubating the disease may succumb. Furthermore, some researchers do not suggest to vaccinate the animals against PPR with TCRP vaccine as there is a chance that PPR virus may mutate and result in evolution of a new variant of PPR virus. So, both the inactivated and lives attenuated vaccines against PPR have been developed. Inactivated PPR vaccine is not suitable as immunity following its use is short lived. Live attenuated Vero cell adapted PPR vaccine developed by IVRI and TNUVAS have been proved to be effective against PPR in sheep and goat. Vaccinia virus recombinants expressing the fusion (vRF) or the haemagglutinin (vRH) and a double recombinant expressing both the genes (vRFH) of RP virus provided complete protection to goats against PPR. The recombinant vaccine using capripox viruses for expression of the fusion and HA protein genes of RP virus also exerted satisfactory level of immunity in goats to be protected against PPR.

Further Reading :

Andreoletti, L., Hober, D., Belaich, S., Lobert, P.E., Dewilde, A. and Wattre, P. (1996). Rapid detection of enterovirus in the clinical specimens using PCR and microwell capture hybridization assat. *J. Virol. Meth.* 62 : 1-10.

Brindha, K., Raj, G.D., Ganesan, P.I., Thiagarajan, V., Nainar, A.M. and Nachimuthu, K. (2001). Comparison of virus isolation and polymerase chain reaction for diagnosis of *Peste des Petits Ruminants*. *Acta Virol.* 45 : 169-172.

Chaudhary, S.S., Pandey, K. D., Singh, R. P., Verma, P. C., and Gupta, P. K. 2009. A Vero cell derived combined vaccine against sheep pox and *Peste des petits ruminants* for sheep. *Vaccine.* 27: 2548-2553.

Dechamma, H.J., Dighe, V., Kumar, Ashok C., Singh, R. P., Jagadish, M. and Kumar, Satish. (2006). Identification of T-helper and Linear B epitope in the hypervariable region of nucleocapsid protein of PPRV and its use in the development of specific antibodies to detect viral antigen. *Vet. Microbiol.* 118: 201-211.

Dhar, P., Muthuchelvan, D., Sanyal, A., Kaul, R., Singh, R.P., Singh, R.K. and Bandyopadhyay, S.K. (2006). Sequence analysis of the haemagglutinin and fusion protein genes of PPR vaccine virus of Indian origin. *Virus Genes.* 32:71-8.

Dhar, P., Sreenivasa, B.P., Bareett, T., Corteyn, M., Singh, R.P. and Bandyopadhyay, S.K. (2002). Recent epidemiology of *Peste des Petits Ruminants virus* (PPRV). *Vet. Microbiol.* 88 : 153-159.

Dhar, P., Sreenivasa, B.P., Barrett, T., Corteyn, M., Singh, R.P. and Bandyopadhyay, S.K. (2002). Recent epidemiology of PPR virus (PPRV). *Vet. Microbiol.* 88(2):153-9.

Diallo, A., Barrett, T., Barbron, M., Shaila, M.S. and Lefvre, P.C. (1989). Differentiation of rinderpest and *Peste des Petits Ruminants* viruses using specific cDNA clones. *J. Virol. Meth.* 23 : 127-136.

Diallo, A., Libeau, G., Couacy-Hymann, E. and Barbron, M. (1995). Recent developments in the diagnosis of rinderpest and *Peste des Petits Ruminants. Vet. Microbiol.* 44 : 307-317.

Forsyth, M.A. and Barrett, T. (1995). Detection and differentiation of rinderpest and *Peste des Petits Ruminants* in diagnostic and experimental samples by PCR using P and F gene specific primers. *Virus Res.* 39 : 151-163.

George, A., Dhar, P., Sreenivasa, B.P., Singh, R.P. and Bandyopadhyay, S.K. (2006). The M and N genes-based simplex and Multiplex PCR are better than the F or H gene-based simplex PCR for PPR virus. *Acta Virol.* 50(4):217-222.

Mondal, B., Sreenivasa, B.P., Dhar, P., Singh, R.P. and Bandyopadhyay, S.K. (2001). Apoptosis induced by peste des petits ruminants virus in goat peripheral blood mononuclear cell. *Virus Res.* 73(2): 113-119.

Muthuchelvan, D., Sanyal, A., Singh, R. P., Hemadri, D., Sen, A., Sreenivasa, B.P., Singh, R.K., and Bandyopadhyay, S. K. (2005). Comparative sequence analysis of the large polymerase protein (L) gene of peste-des-petits ruminants (PPR) vaccine virus of Indian origin. *Arch. Virol.* 150 (12): 2467-2481.

Muthuchelvan, D., Sanyal, A., Sreenivasa, B.P., Saravanan, P., Dhar, P., Singh, R.P., Singh, R.K. and Bandyopadhyay, S.K.(2006). Analysis of the matrix protein gene sequence of the Asian lineage of peste-des-petits ruminants Vaccine virus. *Vet Microbiol.* 113(1-2): 83-7.

Nandi, S. (2004). *Peste des Petits Ruminants* (PPR) in wild animals – a review. In Indian Wildlife Year Book, Vol -3, published by AIZWV, IVRI, Izatnagar and CZA, New Delhi. pp 87-93.

Nandi, S. (2010). Prevalence, diagnosis and immunoprophylaxis of PPR. Lead paper presented in Short Term Training Course on "Laboratory Diagnosis of Animal Diseases and Zoonoses" on 13.12.10 held at Indian Veterinary Research Institute Eastern Regional Station, Kolkata from December 7-20, 2010.

Saravanan, P., Singh, R.P., Balamurugan, V., Dhar, P., Sreenivasa, B.P., Muthuchelvan, D., Sen, A., Aleyas, A.G., Singh, R.K. and Bandyopadhyay, S.K. (2004). Development of a N gene-based PCR-ELISA for detection of Peste-des-petits-ruminants virus in clinical samples. *Acta Virol.* 48(4):249-55.

Sarkar, J., Sreenivasa B.P, Singh R.P., Dhar, P. and Bandyopadhyay S.K. (2003). Comparative efficacy of various chemical stabilizers on the thermostability of live attenuated peste des petits ruminants (PPR) vaccine. *Vaccine.* 21(32): 4728-473.

Shaila, M.S., Purushothaman, V., Bhavasr, D., Venugopal, K. and Venkatesan, R.A. (1989). Peste des Petits Ruminants of sheep in India. *Vet. Rec.* 125 : 602.

Singh, R.P., Sreenivasa, B.P., Dhar, P. and Bandyopadhyay, S.K. (2004). A sandwich ELISA for the diagnosis of *Peste des Petits Ruminants* infection in small ruminants using anti-nucleocapsid protein monoclonal antibody. *Arch. Virol.* 149 : 2155-2170.

Singh, R.P., Sreenivasa, B.P., Dhar, P., Shah, L.C. and Bandyopadhyay, S.K. (2004). Development of a monoclonal antibody based competitive ELISA for detection and titration of antibodies to *Peste des Petits Ruminants virus* (PPRV). *Vet. Microbiol.* 98 : 3-15.

Singh, R.P., Bandyopadhyay, S.K., Sreenivasa, B.P. and Dhar, P. (2004). Production and Characterization of monoclonal antibodies to peste des petits ruminants (PPR) virus. *Vet. Res. Comm.* 28: 623-639.

Singh, R.P., Saravanan, P., Sreenivasa, B.P., Singh, R., K. and Bandyopadhyay S. K. (2004). Prevalence and distribution of peste des petits ruminants (PPR) virus infection in small ruminants of India. *Rev. Sci. Tech. (OIE).* 23 (3): 807-819.

Singh, R.P., Sreenivasa, B.P., Dhar, P., Roy, R.N. and Bandyopadhyay, S.K. (2000). Development of a monoclonal antibody based competitive ELISA for the detection of rinderpest antibodies. *Rev.Sci. Tech. (OIE).* 19 (3): 754-763.

Sreenivasa, B.P., Singh, R.P., Mondal, B., Dhar, P. and Bandyopadhyay, S.K. (2006). Marmoset B95a cells: A sensitive system for cultivation of Peste des Petits Ruminants (PPR) virus. *Vet. Res. Commun.* 30(1):103-8.

❑❑❑

5

Goat Pox

Synonyms : Variola capra

It is a malignant disease of goats characterized by high rise of body temperature and generalized pock lesions.

Distribution : Goat pox has been reported from all parts of the world. Various workers have reported the outbreaks of the disease from different states of India. It is widely prevalent in W.B. and may attain epidemic proportion with mortality rate of 80% in kid and ~50% in adults.

Etiology : The pox virus is one of the largest and most complex of all viruses. There is no nucleocapsid conforming to either of the two types of symmetry found in most of the viruses hence it is called a complex virion. The virus is brick shaped measuring 300X240X100 nm and there is irregular arrangement of tubules on outer membranes. The outer membrane encloses a dumbbell shaped core and two lateral bodies of unknown nature. The core contains the viral DNA together with protein. The causative agent of the goat pox is double stranded DNA containing virus belongs to the genus *Capripox virus,* subfamily *Chordopoxvirinae* and family *Poxviridae.* The nucleic acid is about 200 Kbp in length, has inverted terminal repeats and each end is covalently closed so that on denaturation it forms a large, single stranded circular molecule. The other members of the genus Capripox virus are lumpy skin disease virus and sheep pox virus. Capripox viruses are antigenically and genetically very close to each other. It has been reported that it is possible to infect goats with sheep pox virus and sheep with goat pox virus.

Susceptible hosts : The capripox virus are peculiarly host adapted and are pathogenic only for sheep or goats. Although the Kenyan sheep and goat pox virus strain is the mildest producing only a local lesions in both sheep and goats and local necrotic lesions in cattle. Many strains of Mediterranean regions and from India appear highly adapted to either sheep or goats. Virus strains will produce local reactions when inoculated into the other species and there is no natural cross infection between the two, appears to occur under field condition.

Cattle do not develop any humoral immune response to sheep and goat pox viruses maintained in close contact with infected flocks in Kenya and there is no natural transmission of the virus to cattle.

Sheep pox and goat pox viruses isolated from Scandinavia and India differ in some aspects from the usual forms. A unique property of most of the sheep pox and goat pox virus strains is the high level of host adaptation and inability to infect other animals except man. Small red papules followed by vesicles have been developed on the hands and arms of human beings handling the affected animals, no generalization occurred. The Swedish strain produced lesions in rein deer, and neither any sheep pox strains nor the Kenyan sheep and goat pox virus strain were found to have the zoonotic properties.

None of the wild ungulates in areas where sheep pox and goat pox is in epidemic form has shown antibody to the virus and appeared with skin lesions.

As far as laboratory animals are concerned, they are uniformly refractory to infection to most strains of the virus. The goat strains with pathogenicity for man produce lesions in rabbits and rein deer.

Mode of transmission: The method of transmission of goat pox virus has been the subject of much speculation. The usual mode of transmission is either through contact with infected animal or inhalation. The virus may gain entry through wound and abrasion. The greatest concentrations occur in the skin from 10-14 days and the titre then falls but virus can be detected upto 28 days in necrotic tissue or scabs.The virus may also be transported to other places by dog, cat etc. The disease may be transmitted through food and water mechanically.

Resistance : Goat pox virus like other pox viruses is sensitive to lipid solvent. Most of the pox viruses like orthopox, avipox and leporipox viruses are sensitive to chloform and relatively resistant to diethyl ether, while the sheep pox and goat pox viruses are sensitive to ether. The capripox viruses are acid labile. Like other pox viruses, capripox viruses can survive for the prolonged period in the environment . Goat pox virus in scab material of recovered animal has been shown to be infective for periods of at least 3 months. There is no loss of virus titre in the freeze dried ampoules when kept at -20°C for 5 years.

Pathogenesis : The incubation period is 7-8 days. After getting entry into the body, the virus reaches the blood circulation via lymphatic ducts and is then carried to the skin and target organs. There is development of lung lesions leading to bronchopneumonia. The virus is present in conjunctival and nasal secretions. There is appearance of papules on the mucous membranes. The presence of virus in the skin papules produce irritation and the affected animals rub their body on other animals or walls. There is secondary bacterial infection on skin surface. The virus may pass through placenta to the foetus and pregnant animals may abort.

Clinical signs : The clinical signs of goat pox virus infection vary with different host and in different geographical areas.

Goats of all ages can be affected. The disease is more severe in young animals. The first signs of disease are rhinitis, conjunctivitis and pyrexia (40-42°C). Animals stand with an arched back, have poor body coat and have inappetance. One to two days later, cutaneous lesions develop (0.5-1.5 cm in diameter) often accompanied with lesions on the external nares, lips and within the mouth. The lesions on the skins are largely confined to the areas where the wool or hair is shortest such as on the head, neck, ears, axilla, groin, peritoneum and under the tail.

Lesions present on the tongue and gums tend to ulcerate and high mortality rates occur when lesions develop in the respiratory and alimentary tract. Post-mortem examination shows multiple consolidated areas (0.5-2.0 cm in diameter) in the lungs. Secondary bacterial pneumonia is the common cause of death. Similar lesions are also visible in the liver, kidneys, abomasums and other organs. The appearance of the skin lesions varies and in some outbreaks the lesions are obviously vesicular, they coalesce and involve large areas of the body, especially the lower abdomen.

A nodular form of goat pox has been described in many parts of the world and has been called 'stone pox'. The clinical appearance of the skin lesions is similar to lumpy skin disease.

While lesions may be restricted to predilection sites, they often involve the whole of the body in both young and old animals. Some lesions heal in situ, but the majority form necrotic plugs, which are shed leaving a shallow 'punched out' ulcer. This heals leaving a depressed permanent scar.

When an epidemic occurs in a completely susceptible flock with no previous contact with the virus, the morbidity may be as high as 75% and mortality 50%. Mortality in young animals may approach to 100%.

A sheep and goat pox virus isolate from Kenya is often associated with low morbidity and high level of background immunity (90%). However, a 60% morbidity may be found in areas where there was no previously detectable antibody. Such situation is thought to exists elsewhere and cause very variable figures for morbidity and mortality obtained in different outbreaks.

Clinical management and supportive therapy : All the infected goats should be placed in clean, well ventilated pens and fed on a high plane of nutrition. Animals that are reluctant to feed should be given 10% glucose saline. All the diseased animals should be under the antibiotic coverage (Terramycin injectable solution I/M @ 5 mg/kg body weight) for 5 successive days. The eyes of the affected animals should be washed with 2% boric acid solution and nostrils cleaned and washed with a weak solution of potassium permanganate (1:10,000). Respiration should be stimulated with oleum eucalyptus inhalation or coramine. Terramycin ointment and powder should be applied topically to dry scabby and ulcerated skin lesions.

Lesions : Pock lesions appear in all the parts of the body e.g. nostrils, face, ear, lip, cheek, snout, feet, thigh, abdomen, neck, teat and udder. Papules are formed within 1-3 days. The papules have raised dark brown centres and these changes into vesicles with creamy coloured fluid in 2 days. Skin nodules of varying sizes with thick grey materials are formed within 9-12 days. On 12 days onwards, the nodules regress forming reddish brown crusts which fall off leaving a granulation tissue underneath on 20th days. Lesions are found in the trachea with accompanying catarrhal pneumonia. Lesions occasionally reach abomasums causing haemorrhagic enteritis.

On histological examination the changes comprise of haemorrhages in the epidermis and edema of subcutis. There is ballooning degeneration of epithelial cells, coagulative necrosis with pyknotic nuclei and infiltration of mononuclear cells are evident. The I/C inclusion bodies are observed in the epidermal cells.

Lung parenchyma reveals pneumonic changes characterized by congestion, exudation, thickening of interlobular septa and infiltration of inflammatory cells.

Diagnosis : The disease is diagnosed on the basis of

a) Clinical signs : Pock lesions on the skin throughout the body.

b) Histological examination : I/C inclusion bodies in epidermal cells.

c) Isolation of virus in lamb or kid kidney, testicle cell culture, BHK21 cell line, Vero cell line or chorio-allantoic membrane.

d) AGPT : It gives precipitation bands in 24-48 hours.

e) CIE : It gives precipitation band in 2-3 hours.

f) FAT : Direct FAT is used to detect the presence of pox virus in the oedema fluid. Indirect FAT is employed to determine the antibody status of a flock.

g) ELISA : Immunocapture ELISA can be used to detect the goat pox virus in scab suspension. Indirect ELISA is employed to screen the serum samples for the presence of antibodies against goat pox virus in a flock.

h) Polymerase chain reaction (PCR) : Recently PCR using primers based on the attachment gene has been successfully adopted to detect the capripox virus genomic DNA in skin scab samples. The amplified product could be visualized in phenol-chloroform extracted DNA samples as well as samples which were boiled for 10 minutes only in water bath.

Control

a) Import of animals from disease prone areas are to be prohibited.

b) The destruction of affected flocks or the quarantine of the sick animals from healthy ones.

c) Strict sanitary measures are to be adopted.

d) A killed or BPL inactivated immunoprophylactic agent along with non-specific immunostimulant from *M. phlei* has shown great promise exerting one year protection when administered S/C @ 1 ml/animal.

e) Live attenuated goat pox vaccine adapted and attenuated in cell culture (lamb/kid kidney, testicle, BHK21 , Vero etc) are also available in the market giving solid lifelong protection when administered S/C or I/D @ 1 ml/animal.

Further Reading

Achour, H.A., Bouguedour, R., Bouhbal, A., Guechtouli A. and Aouissat, M. (2000). Comparative study of the immunizing ability of some attenuated strains of sheep pox virus and of a sensitizing vaccine. *Rev. Sci. Tech. (OIE)*. 19 : 773–783.

Bhanuprakash, V., Indrani, B.K., Hegde, R., Kumar, M.M. and Moorthy, A.R.S. (2004). A classical live attenuated vaccine for sheep pox. *Trop. Anim. Hlth Prod.* 36 (4): 307–320.

Bhanuprakash, V., Moorthy, A.R.S., Krishnappa, G., Srinivasa Gowda R.N. and Indrani, B.K. (2003). A live attenuated vaccine for sheep pox, *Indian J. Anim. Sci.* 73 : 1093–1098.

Bhanuprakash, V., Moorthy, A.R.S., Krishnappa, G., Srinivasa Gowda R.N. and Indrani, B.K. (2005). An epidemiological study of sheep pox infection in Karnataka, India. *Rev. Sci. Tech. (OIE).* 24 (3) : 909-920.

Black, D. N., Hammond, J. M. and Kitching, R. P. (1986). Genomic relationship between capripoxviruses. *Virus Res.* 5: 277-292.

Carn, V. M. (1993). Control of capripoxvirus infections. *Vaccine.* 11:1275-1279.

Carn, V. M., Timms, C. P., Chand, P., Black, D. N. and Kitching, R. P. (1994). Protection of goats against capripox using a subunit vaccine. *Vet. Rec.* 135: 434-436.

Carn, V.M. (1995). An antigenic trapping ELISA for the detection of capripox virus in tissue culture supernatant and biopsy samples. *J. Virol. Meth.* **51** : 95–102.

Carn, V.M., Kitching, R.P., Hammond J.M. and Chand, P. (1994). Use of a recombinant antigen in an indirect ELISA for detecting bovine antibody to capripox virus. *J. Virol. Meth.* 49 : 285–294.

Chand, P., Kitching, R.P. and Black, D.N. (1994). Evaluation of the Western blot analysis of virus-specific antibody responses to capripox and contagious pustular dermatitis infections in sheep. *Epidemiol. Infect.* 113(2):377-85

Davies, F. G. (1976). Characteristics of a virus causing a pox disease in sheep and goats in Kenya, with observation on the epidemiology and control. *J. Hyg.* 76: 163-171.

Davies, F. G., and Otema, C. (1981). Relationships of capripox viruses found in Kenya with two Middle Eastern strains and some orthopox viruses. *Res. Vet. Sci.* 31: 253-255.

Diallo, A., Minet, C., Berhe, Le Goff., G. C., Black, D.N. and Fleming, M. (2002). Goat immune response to capripox vaccine expressing the hemagglutinin protein of peste des petits ruminants. *Ann. N.Y. Acad. Sci.* 969 : 88–91.

Garner, M.G., Sawarkar,S.D., Brett, E.K., Edwards, J.R., Kulkarni V.B. and Boyle D.B. (2000). The extent and impact of sheep pox and goat pox in the state of Maharashtra, India. *Trop. Anim. Hlth. Prod.* 32 : 205–223.

Gershon, P. D. and Black, D. N. (1989). The nucleotide sequence around the capripoxvirus thymidine kinase gene reveals a gene shared specifically with leporipoxvirus. *J. Gen. Virol.* 70: 525-533.

Gershon, P. D. and Black, D. N. (1988). A comparison of the genomes of capripoxvirus isolates of sheep, goats, and cattle. *Virology.* 164: 341-349.

Gershon, P. D. and Black, D. N. (1989). A capripoxvirus pseudogene whose only intact homologs are in other poxvirus genomes. *Virology.* 172: 350-354.

Gershon, P. D., Ansell, D. M. and Black, D. N. (1989). A comparison of the genome organization of capripoxvirus with that of the orthopoxviruses. *J. Virol.* 63: 4703-4708.

Gershon, P. D., Kitching, R. P., Hammond, J. M. and Black, D. N. (1989). Poxvirus genetic recombination during natural virus transmission. *J. Gen. Virol.* 70: 485-489.

Heine, H. G., Stevens, M. P., Foord, A. J. and Boyle, D. B. (1999). A capripoxvirus detection PCR and antibody ELISA based on the major antigen P32, the homolog of the vaccinia virus H3L gene. *J. Immunol. Meth.* 227: 187-196.

Hosamani, M., Mondal, B., Tembhurne, P.A., Bandyopadhyay, S.K., Singh, R.K. and Rasool, T.J. (2004). Differentiation of sheep pox and goat poxviruses by sequence analysis and PCR-RFLP of P32 gene. *Virus Gene.* 29 : 73–80.

Hosamani, M., Nandi, S., Mondal, B., Singh, R.K., Rasool T.J. and Bandyopadhyay, S.K. (2004). A vero cell attenuated goat pox virus provides protection against virulent virus challenge. *Acta Virol.* 48: 15–21.

Ireland, D.C. and Binepal, Y.C. (1998). Improved detection of capripoxvirus in biopsy samples by PCR. *J. Virol. Meth.* 74 : 1–7.

Kitching, R. P., and Mellor, P. S. (1986). Insect transmission of capripoxvirus. *Res. Vet. Sci.* 40: 255-258

Kitching, R. P. and Taylor, W. P. (1985). Clinical and antigenic relationship between isolates of sheep and goat pox viruses. *Trop. Anim. Hlth. Prod.* 17: 64-74.

Kitching, R. P., and Taylor, W. P. (1985). Transmission of capripoxvirus. *Res. Vet. Sci.* 39: 196-199.

Kitching, R. P., Bhat, P. P. and Black, D. N. (1989). The characterization of African strains of capripoxvirus. *Epidemiol. Infect.* 102: 335-343.

Kitching, R. P., Hammond, J. M. and Taylor, W. P. (1987). A single vaccine for the control of capripox infection in sheep and goats. *Res. Vet. Sci.* 42: 53-60.

Kitching, R. P., McGrane, J. J. and Taylor, W. P. (1986). Capripox in the Yemen Arab Republic and the Sultanate of Oman. *Trop. Anim. Health Prod.* 18: 115-122.

Kitching, R. P., McGrane, J. J., Hammond, J. M., Miah, A. H., Mustafa, A. H. and Majumder. J. R. (1987). Capripox in Bangladesh. *Trop. Anim. Health Prod.* 19: 203-208.

Kitching, R.P. (2003). Vaccines for lumpy skin disease, sheep pox and goat pox. *Dev. Biol.* 114: 161–167.

Kotwal, G. J., and Moss, B. (1988). Analysis of a large cluster of nonessential genes deleted from a vaccinia virus terminal transposition mutant. *Virology.* 167: 524-537.

Mangana-Vougiouka, O., Martoulatos, P., Koptopoulos, G., Nomikou, K., Bakandritsos N. and Papadopoulos, O. (2000). Sheep poxvirus identification from clinical specimens by PCR, cell culture, immunofluorescence and agar gel immunoprecipitation assay. *Mol. Cell Probe.* 14 : 305–310.

Munz, E., and Dumbell, K. (1994). Sheep pox and goat pox, p. 613-615. *In* J. A. W. Coetzer, G. R. Thomson, and R. C. Tustin (ed.), Infectious diseases of livestock, vol. 1. Oxford University Press, Cape Town, South Africa.

Nandi, S. and Rao, T.V.S. (1997). Goat pox – a major threat to goat industry in India. *Indian Farming.* 47: 3: 26-27.

Ngichabe, C. K., Wamwayi, H. M., Barrett, T., Ndungu, E. K., Black, D. N. and Bostock, C. J. (1997). Trial of a capripoxvirus-rinderpest recombinant vaccine in African cattle. *Epid. Infect.* 118: 63-70.

O.I.E. (2000) Manual of standards for diagnostic tests and vaccines (4th ed) (2000) [chapter 2.1.10].

Ramprabhu, R., Priya, W.S.S., Chandran, N.D.J., Mohan, A.C. and Prathaban, S.(2002). Clinical, hematological, epidemiological and virological studies in two sheep pox outbreaks. Indian J. Small Ruminants. 8(2): 129–130.

Rao, T. V., and Bandyopadhyay, S. K. (2000). A comprehensive review of goat pox and sheep pox and their diagnosis. *Anim. Hlth. Res. Rev.* 1: 127-136.

Sadhukhan, T., Nag, N.C., Ray, J.P., Nandi, S. and Das, R. (1998). Application of dot-ELISA in the diagnosis of goat pox outbreak. *Indian Vet. J.* 75: 841-842.

Singh, I.P., Pandey R. and Srivastava, R.N. (1979). Sheep pox: a review. *Vet. Bull.* 49 : (3): 145–154.

Tiwari, A.K., Negi, B.S., Roy, R.N. and Nandi, S. (1995). Comparative evaluation of dot-ELISA and RPHA in the diagnosis of goat pox. *Indian Vet. Med. J.* 19:4:266-268.

Tiwari, A.K., Nandi, S. and Negi, B.S. (1995). Reverse phase passive haemagglutination (RPHA) test for the detection of goat pox virus antigen. *Indian J. Virol.* 11:2:35-37.

Tulman, E.R., Afimo, C.L., Lu, Z., Zsak, L., Sur J.H. and Sandybaev N.T. (2002). The genomes of sheep pox and goat poxviruses. *J. Virol.* 76 : 12 : 6054–6061.

Yeruham, I., Perl, S., Nyska, A., Abraham, A., Davidson, M., Haymovitch, M., Zamir, O. and Grinstein, H. (1994). Adverse reactions in cattle to a capripox vaccine. *Vet. Rec.* 135: 330-332.

6

Sheep Pox

Synonyms : Variola ovine, ovine pox

Sheep pox causes a severe and highly contagious disease in sheep which is listed in group A disease of the OIE. It is defined as a malignant pox of sheep characterized by fever and generalized development of pock lesions. Lesions first appear as vesicles which later turn into pustules on the exposed parts of the body. There is high mortality rate in lambs.

Distribution : The disease is in existence since very long in Asia and Europe. It is prevalent in many areas of middle East countries, Africa, Asia and Mediterranean countries. There are lot of disease outbreaks in India around the year. European Union with the exception of occasional sporadic outbreak in eastern areas of Greece, U.S.A. and Australia are free from the disease.

Etiology : The pox virus is one of the largest and most complex of all viruses. There is no nucleocapsid conforming to either of the two types of symmetry found in most of the viruses hence it is called a complex virion. The virus is brick shaped measuring 300X240X100 nm and there is irregular arrangement of tubules on outer membranes. The outer membrane encloses a dumbbell shaped core and two lateral bodies of unknown nature. The core contains the viral DNA together with protein. The causative agent of the sheep pox is double stranded DNA containing virus belongs to the genus *Capripox virus*, subfamily *Chordopoxvirinae* and family *Poxviridae.* The nucleic acid is about 200 Kbp in length, has inverted terminal repeats and each end is covalently closed so that on denaturation it forms a large, single stranded circular molecule. The other members of the genus Capripox virus are lumpy skin disease virus and goat pox virus. Capripox viruses are antigenically and genetically very close to each other. It has been reported that it is possible to infect goats with sheep pox virus and sheep with goat pox virus.

Susceptible hosts : The sheep are naturally susceptible. The susceptibility also depends on the breed and age of animals. Younger sheep are more susceptible over older ones. In young lambs, the disease may flare up in epidemic proportion. Merino breed is more susceptible over indigenous one.

Transmission : The disease spreads by direct or indirect contact with contaminated objects. In infected pens, the scab virus can remain viable for as long as 6 months. Infection can occur through either the respiratory or the cutaneous route. Mechanical transmission by arthropods may occur. Affected sheep shed the virus at every stage of the disease up to 8 weeks after the lesions have healed. Merino sheep are most susceptible whereas Algerian sheep are comparatively resistant. On inhalation, the virus enters the lungs where from it enters the circulation by lymphatic channels and is then carried to skin and mucous membranes. The virus may pass from the infected ewe to the foetus through placental blood and the lambs may be born with pox lesions.

Pathogenesis : On entrance , there is multiplication of the virus and resultant viraemia. The virus get distributed throughout the body system and generalized skin infection takes place. There is infiltration of cells and necrosis of the epidermal layers. Prickle cell layers of the skin proliferate and this extends to the corium. Vesicles thus appear are multilobular in nature. Vesicles turn into scabs. Intracytoplasmic acidophilic inclusion bodies are present in the infected epithelial cells. The virus may affect mucous membrane of the pharynx, trachea, and abomasums. There is formation of vesicles and ulcers but inflammatory changes are occasionally noticed in intestinal and respiratory tract mucosa. The incubation period varies from 4 to 14 days.

Clinical signs : The clinical signs of sheep pox depends on the breed of sheep, the virulence of the virus strain, the nature of secondary infection and organ involved. The disease may appear usually in three different clinical forms. (a) Malignant form (b) Mild (benign) form and (c) Abortive form.

(a) Malignant form : This is the most common form. It is characterized first by appearance of marked general distress with elevated high temperature (106-107°F), rough staring coat, loss of appetite and numerous areas of erythema all over the body surface. The eruptions are more prominent on the cheeks, nostrils, lips, ears, eyelids, vulva, armpits, thighs, chest, mammary glands, testicles and under surface of the tail. The lesions pass through the typical pock stages. The vesicular stage which may be haemorrhagic with a tendency to generalize, is followed by the development of pustules which later turn into scabs. Healing is slow and may take more than a month. Approximately 35-40% of the affected cases develop secondary pneumonia characterized by respiratory distress, cough and thick mucopurulent nasal discharge. Such cases are invariably terminated fatally and profuse watery diarrhea of foetid nature with sub-normal body temperature before death is almost a constant feature. Affected animals may also die of disease due to pyaemia or septicaemia caused by secondary bacterial complications.

(b) Mild (benign) form : Adult Algerian and indigenous sheep are usually affected with this form and eruptions are confined around eyes, lips and nose.

(c) Abortive form : Generalization is rare and mortality is low (5%). Ewe may abort foetus with pock lesions. Lactating ewe may develop the signs of mastitis due to lesions in the udder.

Pathology : The characteristic papules, vesicles, pustules and scabs are noted on cutaneous surface. Numerous circular nodules grayish white in colour and comparatively of smaller diameter (4-6 mm) than those of the skin are always present throughout the tissues of the lungs. Consolidation of apical, cardiac and ventro-lateral borders of the diaphragmatic lobes with marked oedema is present in about 35% cases. The reddish fluid oozes out on cutting the oedematous lungs. The pleura show no gross lesions. The trachea shows petechial haemorrhages with few ulcers and purulent exudates.

The petechial haemorrhages are found on epicardium and endocardium of the heart. The liver is found enlarged and acutely congested. The kidneys are usually affected with white infarcts and subscapular haemorrhages and showed intense congestion of both medulla and cortex. Adrenals are also congested.

No gross lesion is seen in the muscles, body fat, peritoneum, spleen, pancreas, thymus, thyroid, uterus, vagina, brain, spinal cord, bones and bone marrow. The mediastinal, mesenteric and prescapular lymph glands are usually enlarged and oedematous.

Diagnosis

Presumptive diagnosis : This is based on characteristic lesions on the skin. Intracytoplasmic acidophilic inclusion bodies are observed in the infected cells under histopathological studies.

Confirmatory diagnosis : A number of serological tests, viz., complement fixation test, immunodiffusion test, counterimmunoelectrophoresis test, spot agglutination test, reverse phase passive haemagglutination test, single radial haemolysis test, enzyme linked immunosorbent assay and dot- enzyme linked immunosorbent assay are available for the detection of sheep pox virus antigen and antibody. Besides, the sheep pox can be diagnosed by inoculating the lymph or skin materials of the affected sheep on the scarified skin of the suspected animal which will show rise of temperature, characteristic papules, vesicles and pustules. Secondary pox lesions will appear on abdomen, thighs, eyelids and ears. Recently Polymerase chain reaction (PCR) using primers based on the attachment gene has been successfully adopted to detect the capripox virus genomic DNA in skin scab samples. The amplified product could be visualized in phenol-chloroform extracted DNA sample as well as samples which were boiled for 10 minutes only in water bath.

Differential diagnosis : It should be differentiated from bluetongue and contagious ecthyma.

Clinical management and supportive therapy : All the infected sheep should be placed in clean, well ventilated house and fed on a high level of balanced nutrition. Animals reluctant to feed should be given 10% glucose saline perenterally. All the diseased animals should be under the antibiotic coverage (5 mg/kg body weight Terramycin injectable solution I/M for 5 successive days) to restrict the secondary bacterial infections. The eyes of the animals should be washed with 2% boric acid solution and nostrils cleaned and washed with a weak solution of potassium permanganate (1:10 000). Respiration should be stimulated with oleum eucalyptus inhalation or coramine. Terramycin ointment and powder should be applied topically to dry scabby and ulcerated skin lesions.

Control : Vaccines being the most economical and efficient way to control and eradicate a disease has been proved in several other viral diseases. A variety of vaccines both inactivated and live attenuated have been developed since the beginning of the century by a number of researchers employing aluminium hydroxide, alum and saponin as adjuvant and formalin, merthiolate and BPL as inactivating agent. The route of administration of most of the vaccines is either I/D, S/C or I/M and elicited an immune response lasted for 6 months to 1 year. However, in India now-a-days live attenuated tissue culture sheep pox vaccines are mainly produced by two manufacturers, viz., IVRI, Izatnagar and Biomed, U.P. The details of the vaccine is as follows.

Defintion : It is a live attenuated freeze dried vaccine which confers immunity in all breeds of sheep against sheep pox. The vaccine evokes thermal and/or local cutaneous reaction following vaccination without generalization.

Reconstitution : The content of each freeze dried ampoule should be reconstituted in cold sterile normal saline as per the doses indicated on the label. It should be used within 2 hours of reconstitution.

Dose : 0.1 ml for all age groups, I/D in the caudal fold. It can also be inoculated on the tip of the ear.

Immunity : The vaccine is expected to provide immunity for about 1 year.

Storage : The vaccine can be stored at 2-4°C for 3 months.

Note :

(i) All the sheep in the enzootic area should be regularly vaccinated every year. In case of breakdown of immunity the reason must be investigated.

(ii) Lambs or sheep not showing 'take' following vaccination should be revaccinated.

(iii) In few cases, where local reaction progresses to ulceration application of boroglycerine is suggested to alleviate the condition.

Sheep pox is enzootic in India. About 250 outbreaks affecting about one third of total sheep population are reported in India every year causing enormous losses. As sheep rearing is mostly the livelihood of small and marginal farmers in the rural areas, the importance of the disease is clearly revealed. So, to control the disease, the prudent approach is the regular immunization of all the susceptible flocks with a potent and efficacious vaccine. Besides, proper monitoring and stringent surveillance of the disease should be carried out in regular interval to get a clear picture of the disease in India. Lastly, proper management, hygienic condition, sanitation and balanced ration should be provided along with the other measures to keep the disease under control.

Further reading

Achour, H.A., Bouguedour, R., Bouhbal, A., Guechtouli A. and Aouissat, M. (2000). Comparative study of the immunizing ability of some attenuated strains of sheep pox virus and of a sensitizing vaccine. *Rev. Sci. Tech. (OIE).* 19 : 773–783.

Bhanuprakash, V., Indrani, B.K., Hegde, R., Kumar, M.M. and Moorthy, A.R.S. (2004). A classical live attenuated vaccine for sheep pox. *Trop. Anim. Hlth Prod.* 36 (4): 307–320.

Bhanuprakash, V., Moorthy, A.R.S., Krishnappa, G., Srinivasa Gowda R.N. and Indrani, B.K. (2003). A live attenuated vaccine for sheep pox. *Indian J. Anim. Sci.* 73 : 1093–1098.

Bhanuprakash, V., Moorthy, A.R.S., Krishnappa, G., Srinivasa Gowda R.N. and Indrani, B.K. (2005). An epidemiological study of sheep pox infection in Karnataka, India. *Rev. Sci. Tech. (OIE).* 24 (3) : 909-920.

Black, D. N., Hammond, J. M. and Kitching, R. P. (1986). Genomic relationship between capripoxviruses. *Virus Res.* 5: 277-292.

Carn, V. M. (1993). Control of capripoxvirus infections. *Vaccine.* 11:1275-1279.

Carn, V. M., Timms, C. P., Chand, P., Black, D. N. and Kitching, R. P. (1994). Protection of goats against capripox using a subunit vaccine. *Vet. Rec.* 135: 434-436.

Carn, V.M. (1995). An antigenic trapping ELISA for the detection of capripox virus in tissue culture supernatant and biopsy samples. *J. Virol. Meth.* 51 : 95–102.

Carn, V.M., Kitching, R.P., Hammond J.M. and Chand, P. (1994). Use of a recombinant antigen in an indirect ELISA for detecting bovine antibody to capripox virus. *J. Virol. Meth.* 49 : 285–294.

Chand, P., Kitching, R.P. and Black, D.N. (1994). Evaluation of the Western blot analysis of virus-specific antibody responses to capripox and contagious pustular dermatitis infections in sheep. *Epidemiol. Infect.* 113(2) :377-85

Davies, F. G. (1976). Characteristics of a virus causing a pox disease in sheep and goats in Kenya, with observation on the epidemiology and control. *J. Hyg.* 76: 163-171.

Davies, F. G., and Otema, C. (1981). Relationships of capripox viruses found in Kenya with two Middle Eastern strains and some orthopox viruses. *Res. Vet. Sci.* 31: 253-255.

Diallo, A., Minet, C., Berhe, Le Goff., G. C., Black, D.N. and Fleming, M. (2002). Goat immune response to capripox vaccine expressing the hemagglutinin protein of peste des petits ruminants. *Ann. N.Y. Acad. Sci.* 969 : 88–91.

Garner, M.G., Sawarkar,S.D., Brett, E.K., Edwards, J.R., Kulkarni V.B. and Boyle D.B. (2000). The extent and impact of sheep pox and goat pox in the state of Maharashtra, India. *Trop. Anim. Hlth. Prod.* 32 : 205–223.

Gershon, P. D. and Black, D. N. (1989). The nucleotide sequence around the capripoxvirus thymidine kinase gene reveals a gene shared specifically with leporipoxvirus. *J. Gen. Virol.* 70: 525-533.

Gershon, P. D. and Black, D. N. (1988). A comparison of the genomes of capripoxvirus isolates of sheep, goats, and cattle. *Virology.* 164: 341-349.

Gershon, P. D. and Black, D. N. (1989). A capripoxvirus pseudogene whose only intact homologs are in other poxvirus genomes. *Virology.* 172: 350-354.

Gershon, P. D., Ansell, D. M. and Black, D. N. (1989). A comparison of the genome organization of capripoxvirus with that of the orthopoxviruses. *J. Virol.* 63: 4703-4708.

Gershon, P. D., Kitching, R. P., Hammond, J. M. and Black, D. N. (1989). Poxvirus genetic recombination during natural virus transmission. *J. Gen. Virol.* 70: 485-489.

Heine, H. G., Stevens, M. P., Foord, A. J. and Boyle, D. B. (1999). A capripoxvirus detection PCR and antibody ELISA based on the major antigen P32, the homolog of the vaccinia virus H3L gene. *J. Immunol. Meth.* 227: 187-196.

Hosamani, M., Mondal, B., Tembhurne, P.A., Bandyopadhyay, S.K., Singh, R.K. and Rasool, T.J. (2004). Differentiation of sheep pox and goat poxviruses by sequence analysis and PCR-RFLP of P32 gene. *Virus Gene.* 29 : 73–80.

Hosamani, M., Nandi, S., Mondal, B., Singh, R.K., Rasool T.J. and Bandyopadhyay, S.K. (2004). A vero cell attenuated goat pox virus provides protection against virulent virus challenge. *Acta Virol.* 48: 15–21.

Ireland, D.C. and Binepal, Y.C. (1998). Improved detection of capripoxvirus in biopsy samples by PCR. *J. Virol. Meth.* 74 : 1–7.

Kitching, R. P., and Mellor, P. S. (1986). Insect transmission of capripoxvirus. *Res. Vet. Sci.* 40: 255-258

Kitching, R. P. and Taylor, W. P. (1985). Clinical and antigenic relationship between isolates of sheep and goat pox viruses. *Trop. Anim. Hlth. Prod.* 17: 64-74.

Kitching, R. P., and Taylor, W. P. (1985). Transmission of capripoxvirus. *Res. Vet. Sci.* 39: 196-199.

Kitching, R. P., Bhat, P. P. and Black, D. N. (1989). The characterization of African strains of capripoxvirus. *Epidemiol. Infect.* 102: 335-343.

Kitching, R. P., Hammond, J. M. and Taylor, W. P. (1987). A single vaccine for the control of capripox infection in sheep and goats. *Res. Vet. Sci.* 42: 53-60.

Kitching, R. P., McGrane, J. J. and Taylor, W. P. (1986). Capripox in the Yemen Arab Republic and the Sultanate of Oman. *Trop. Anim. Hlth. Prod.* 18: 115-122.

Kitching, R. P., McGrane, J. J., Hammond, J. M., Miah, A. H., Mustafa, A. H. and Majumder. J. R. (1987). Capripox in Bangladesh. *Trop. Anim. Hlth. Prod.* 19: 203-208.

Kitching, R.P. (2003). Vaccines for lumpy skin disease, sheep pox and goat pox. *Dev. Biol.* 114: 161–167.

Kotwal, G. J., and Moss, B. (1988). Analysis of a large cluster of nonessential genes deleted from a vaccinia virus terminal transposition mutant. *Virology.* 167: 524-537.

Mangana-Vougiouka, O., Martoulatos, P., Koptopoulos, G., Nomikou, K., Bakandritsos N. and Papadopoulos, O. (2000). Sheep poxvirus identification from clinical specimens by PCR, cell culture, immunofluorescence and agar gel immunoprecipitation assay. *Mol. Cell Probe.* 14 : 305–310.

Munz, E., and Dumbell, K. (1994). Sheep pox and goat pox, p. 613-615. *In* J. A. W. Coetzer, G. R. Thomson, and R. C. Tustin (ed.), Infectious diseases of livestock, vol. 1. Oxford University Press, Cape Town, South Africa.

Ngichabe, C. K., Wamwayi, H. M., Barrett, T., Ndungu, E. K., Black, D. N. and Bostock, C. J. (1997). Trial of a capripoxvirus-rinderpest recombinant vaccine in African cattle. *Epid. Infect.* 118: 63-70.

O.I.E. (2000). Manual of standards for diagnostic tests and vaccines (4th ed) (2000) [chapter 2.1.10].

Ramprabhu, R., Priya, W.S.S., Chandran, N.D.J., Mohan, A.C. and Prathaban, S.(2002). Clinical, hematological, epidemiological and virological studies in two sheep pox outbreaks. *Indian J. Small Ruminants.* 8(2): 129–130.

Rao, T.V.S., Malik, Poonam., Nandi, S., Negi, B.S. (1997). Evaluation of immunocapture ELISA for diagnosis of goat pox. *Acta Virologica*. 41 : 345-348.

Rao, T. V., and Bandyopadhyay, S. K. (2000). A comprehensive review of goat pox and sheep pox and their diagnosis. *Anim. Hlth. Res. Rev.* 1: 127-136.

Singh, I.P., Pandey R. and Srivastava, R.N. (1979). Sheep pox: a review. *Vet. Bull.* 49 : (3): 145–154.

Tulman, E.R., Afimo, C.L., Lu, Z., Zsak, L., Sur, J.H. and Sandybaev, N.T. (2002). The genomes of sheep pox and goat poxviruses. *J. Virol.* 76 : 12 : 6054–6061.

Yeruham, I., Perl, S., Nyska, A., Abraham, A., Davidson, M., Haymovitch, M., Zamir, O. and Grinstein, H. (1994). Adverse reactions in cattle to a capripox vaccine. *Vet. Rec.* 135: 330-332.

7

Bluetongue

Synonyms : Catarrhal fever, Sore mouth, Epizootic catarrh, Sore muzzle, Pseudo foot and mouth disease, Malarial catarrhal fever.

It is an infectious, noncontagious arthropod borne viral disease of domestic and wild ruminants namely sheep, goat , cattle, camels, llamas, deer and antelopes. This is predominantly a disease of sheep but occasionally cattle and goats are subclinically affected. The disease is characterized by high fever, catarrhal stomatitis, rhinitis, enteritis and lameness due to inflammation of the coronary bands and sensitive laminae of the feet. There are at least 25 serotypes of bluetongue virus worldwide within the BTV serogroup. Genetic variability occurs within a group due to genetic drift of individual gene segments and genetic reassortment when ruminants or other vectors are infected with more than one strain.

Bluetongue (BT) is now established as endemic disease of animals in India. Antibodies against a number of serotypes of bluetongue virus have been detected in sheep, goat , cattle , buffalo in different parts of the country. The BT disease has been included in OIE list A which has resulted in strict quarantine measures and expensive and costly testing.

Distribution : BT disease remained confined to African continent for nearly 50 years after it's first report by Hutcheon (1902). Cyprus is the first country outside Africa to report BT followed by Turkey (1954), Israel (1951), USA (1952) and Spain (1957). The virus was first isolated in USA from cases of 'Sore muzzle' in sheep in cell culture system. A major epizootic of bluetongue (BTV-10) occurred in Portugal and Spain in 1956-1957, which killed 1,79,000 sheep with a mortality rate of 5%. In Australia, BTV was first isolated from an insect vector in 1977. In the Indian subcontinent, the disease was first reported from West Pakistan (now Pakistan) in 1959 in a flock of Ramboullet sheep imported from USA. In India, the disease was first reported among sheep and goats of Maharashtra state based on clinical signs and detection of BTV specific antibody in sera of recovered animal by Sapre. Later BT was reported from several states like Uttar Pradesh, Haryana, Andhra Pradesh, Rajasthan, Karnataka, Gujarat, M.P. etc on the basis of virus isolation in chicken embryo or cell culture system. BT virus has also been isolated from Culicoides species.

Etiology : The disease is caused by a double stranded RNA virus belonging to the genus *Orbivirus* and family *Reoviridae*. The virus genome of 10 ds RNA segments of varying lengths with a total length of 23 kbp which code for the 7 structural and 4 non-structural proteins. The BT virus is non-enveloped, spherical and about 70 nm of diameter. The virions contain two icosahedral protein shells termed as inner core and indistinct outer capsid. Upon removal of outer capsid protein layer, the virion is converted into the core particle which is 58-60 nm in diameter. The inner capsid or core is a stable structure consisting of 32 capsomeres arranged in icosahedral symmetry. The characteristic ring like configuration leads to the name of this Orbivirus (Orbi meaning ring or circle).

There are seven structural proteins and four non-structural (NS) proteins. The structural proteins are numbered as VP1 to VP7 in order of decreasing size based on electrophoretic migration in SDS-PAGE. The nonstructural proteins are designated as NS1, NS2, NS3 and NS3A. The outer capsid of BTV consists of two major polypeptides i.e. VP2 and VP5, which together constitute approximately 40% of the total BTV protein. Both VP2 and VP5 are attached to the core particle (VP7), although it has been reported that VP5 is more closely associated with the core particle than VP2. VP2 and VP5 show the largest variation in size among the structural proteins of the different BTV serotypes. Further peptide mapping indicates that VP2 is unique for each of the BTV serotypes, where as VP5 revealed an intermediate level of conservation. The variability of VP2 and VP5 protein reflects the role of these proteins in the induction of serotype specific neutralizing antibody. The outer capsid proteins are associated with the virulence and cell adsorption and VP2 is a haemagglutinating protein.

The BTV core is composed of 2 major polypeptides (VP3 and VP7) and 3 minor polypeptides (VP1, VP4 and VP6). The surface of core particle consists entirely of 780 copies of VP7. Beneath the VP7 layer, the sub core is composed of 120 copies of VP3 which encloses the 10 linear ds RNA segments and 3 minor proteins on VP1, VP4 and VP6. VP7 has been identified as the soluble group specific antigen. Among the nonstructural proteins, NS1 and NS2 are identified as major and NS3 and NS3A as minor non-structural proteins respectively.

Susceptible hosts : Although all the domesticated and wild ruminants are susceptible to bluetongue disease, it is basically a disease of sheep. Young sheep under 1 year are more prone to infection. British and Merino sheep are more susceptible than African sheep. European mutton breeds are more susceptible than the Merino. Frank clinical cases of bluetongue were not detected in indigenous (Nali and Sondi) and cross bred sheep indicating that they are comparatively more resistant to bluetongue virus. The disease remains in subclinical form in cattle but cattle may show overt clinical signs with high mortality rate. The degree of susceptibility of goats, although variable, is markedly less than that of sheep. White tailed deer and other wild ruminants may be naturally infected.

Epidemiology : Bluetongue virus causes serious disease in sheep but little or subclinical illness in cattle, buffalo and goat. Under natural condition the viral infection is common in sheep, cattle, elk, white tailed deer, pronghorn antelope, camels and other ruminants. It is interesting to note that deer can be infected by bluetongue or epizootic haemorrhagic disease of deer or both. The diseases are very similar and the viruses are also similar but distinguishable serologically and in culture in chick embryos. Both the viruses have also been isolated from cattle. The BT virus has been isolated from cattle as long as 81 days after infection. Exposure to sunlight and environmental stress appear to increase the severity of the disease.

The morbidity rate varies with the size of the insect population and the immune status of the sheep. If a flock is affected for the first time, morbidity may reach 50-75% and the mortality 20-50%.

The disease can be transmitted experimentally by the inoculation of infective blood but under natural conditions it appear to be spread only by insect bites. Vectors for BT virus are sand flies (*Culicoides sp.*), *Aedes lineatopennis* and *Melophagus ovinus*. The argasid tick *Ornithodoros coriaecells* has been shown experimentally to be capable of transmitting the virus. *Culicoides sp.* do not become infective until about 10 days after ingesting infective blood. *Melophagus ovinus* can transmit the virus in a mechanical manner.

The disease is not spread by contact and there is a marked seasonal incidence during late summer and early autumn when the environment for vector multiplication is congenial. The disease is most prevalent in wet and low lying areas, conditions which favours insect multiplification.

Recovered animals are considered to be reservoir of infection and thus act as carrier of the virus from one season to other. Virus has been isolated from recovered sheep 4 months and from cattle 49 days after infection. The virus has been observed in the semen of the infected bulls and infection is transmitted from infected to healthy cows by insemination. Evidence of vertical transmission from infected dam to offspring has been described but does not generally occur.

Mode of transmission : Bluetongue virus is transmitted by *culicoides species* and is only enzootic in areas where adults of competent vector species are present for most of the time of the year, thus maintaining a continuous series of virus. The species of culicoides which are known to act as vectors for bluetongue virus are most active in the temperature range of 18-29°C and almost inactive below 10°C or above 30°C. There are in excess of 1000 species of culicoides worldwide, only six are known to be capable of transmitting the virus. These include *C. variipennis, C. imicola, C. filvus, C. actoni, C. wadai and* C. *nubeculosus.*

The geographic and seasonal distribution of vectors is critical for both the spread and maintenance of the bluetongue virus in the field. At ambient temperature of 25°C, productive infection in the salivary glands and the ability to transmit the virus, takes approximately seven days after ingesion of the original viraemic blood meal. Only females of the culicoides vectors take blood meal from vertebrate hosts prior to egg laying. Exposure to sun rays seems to increase the severity of infection. The disease is more prevalent in late summer and early autumn which makes congenial environment for the multiplication of the vectors.

White tailed deer and antelope are considered to be reservoir of infection and thus act as carrier of virus from one season to other. The virus has also been detected in the semen of infected bull.

Pathogenesis : On entrance through the bite of the vector, the virus multiplies in the blood stream and leads to a primary viraemic stage. The virus has an affinity for the endothelium, precapillary arterioles, venules and red blood cells. Small vessels underlying stratified squamous epithelium, particularly the oral mucous membrane, skin and coronet of the hoof are mostly affected. The virus is also detected in reculoendothelial cells of lymph nodes especially those draining tissue of the head. The characteristic lesions appear due to damage of blood vessels. It produces hyperemia, haemorrhages and oedema of various tissue. Bluetongue disease is generally more severe in recently shorn than in unshorn sheep. The virus has got both abortigenic and teratogenic characteristics.

Clinical signs : The disease is divided into 3 forms (a) acute (b) subacute and (c) chronic. Naturally occurring acute bluetongue disease in sheep has an incubation period of less than a week (2-4 days in experimentally infected sheep). There is high rise of temperature (105-106°C), nasal discharge, salivation and lacrymation. The nasal discharge is mucopurulent and often blood stained and the saliva is frothy. Swelling and edema of the lips, gums, dental pad and tongue may be evident. There may be ulceration of the lips, dental pad, gum and tongue. Necrotic ulcers develops on the lateral aspects of the tongue which is swollen and purple in colour hence the disease is called bluetongue. Foot lesions including laminitis and coronitis and manifested by lameness and recumbency appear when the mouth lesions begins to heal. The appearance of a dark red to purple band in the skin just above the coronet is considered to be an important diagnostic sign. The twisting of head and neck to one side (wryneck) may be seen in few cases about 12 th day. Oedema of the face, jaws and the ears and hyperemia of the wool less skin may be present. Diarrhoea and dysentery may supervene. Rapid shallow respiration is not uncommon and pneumonia may be evident.

Subacute or subclinical form is noticed in cattle and goats. There is a mild to moderate fever, hyperemia of the mucosa and conjunctiva. Some cattle may develop syndrome like that seen in severely affected sheep. This form of the disease in cattle appears to be a hypersensitivity reaction in a previously affected animal. The same hypersensitivity does not occur in sheep.

Cattle and sheep infected during early pregnancy may cause abortion of congenital deformities which include hydranencephaly , microcephaly, curvature of the limbs, blindness and deformity of the jaw.

Course : In mild cases, the prognosis is generally favourable and recovery is usually rapid and uneventful with some loss of condition. In severe cases , the prognosis should be guarded. Animals which appear to be recovering satisfactorily may suddenly collapse and die. On the other hand, animals which have had severe symptoms may recover completely. The recovery is usually prolonged when animals are weak and debilitated because of varying degree of buccal lesions and muscular involvement. Lambs especially take a long time to recover and usually remain runts.

The mortality rate in bluetongue varies remarkably and the outcome is influenced by various factors. The pathogenicity of virus strains differs markedly and the sunlight is known to aggravate the clinical course of the disease. The disease is more severe in recently shorn sheep than in sheep with long fleeces. When sheep exposed suboptimally to bluetongue virus followed by challenged intradermally with the same virus showed more severe clinical reactions than sheep inoculated intradermally only, the phenomenon is called virus sensitization or increased susceptibility to bluetongue virus.

Under field conditions. The mortality rate usually varies between 2-30%. Death occurs mostly from 1-8 days after the appearance of visible signs. Bronchopneumonia often resulting from aspiration of rumen ingesta, is probably the most common cause of death.

Pathology : The severity and distribution of the lesions found in bluetongue infected sheep depend on the severity of the clinical symptoms and particular state of the disease at which death occurs. The typical pathological picture may be largely obscured by secondary complications such as bronchopneumonia or metabolic disturbances in animals dying late in the course of the disease.

The prominent lesions of digestive system are usually found in and around the mouth. The mucosa is oedematous, hyperemic and cyanotic and petechiae or ecchymoses may be present. Excoriations are evident on the lips, dental pads, anterior dorsum of the tongue and internal surface of the cheek. The excoriation are covered with grey necrotic tissue. Hyperemia of the ruminal papillae, ruminal pillars and reticular folds is commonly observed. The remainder of the digestive tract may show congestion and catarrhal inflammation.

In the respiratory system the nose is frequently partly occluded by a grayish brown scab composed of desquamated epithelium, inspissated serum and foreign debris. The trachea may contain white forth and the lungs may be oedematous and pneumonia is common as a result of inhalation of ingesta.

In cardiovascular system, there is widespread hyperaemia, oedema and haemorrrhages. Distinctive haemorrhages, ranging in size from 2 to 15 mm are consistently found at the base of the pulmonary artery and are generally considered as pathognomic of bluetongue. Subepicardial haemorrhages near the apex of the heart and subendocardial haemorrhages on the papillary muscles may be present. Petechiae are observed in the pericardium along with mild hydropericardium and hydrothorax.

The lymph nodes, particular those draining tissues of the head are commonly enlarged, oedematous and haemorrhagic. The spleen may be slightly enlarged and subscapular petechial haemorrhages may be present in the thymus.

The lesions in the skeletal muscles mostly observed in thigh, shoulder, back and neck consist of petechial or ecchymotic haemorrhages and hyaline degeneration. The muscular degeneration continued even the subsidence of fever and is largely responsible for the severe emaciation characteristic of bluetongue.

The kidneys are commonly congested with petechial haemorrhages on the mucosa of the urinary bladder, urethra, vulva or penile sheath.

Diagnosis : Presumptive diagnosis : It is based on the history, clinical findings (oedematous swelling and cyanosis), seasonal occurrence and negation of spread by direct contact.

Confirmatory diagnosis : The serological tests which are generally used for confirmatory diagnosis of bluetongue consist of agar gel diffusion test, plaque inhibition test, neutralization test, fluorescent antibody test, complement fixation test, ELISA and dot-ELISA. Besides, isolation of bluetongue virus in suitable system viz., sheep, chicken embryo or cell culture inoculation offer the alternative method of confirmatory diagnosis. Recently molecular biological techniques viz., RT-PCR based on the structural protein and nonstructural protein gene specific primers, nucleic acid hybridization and nucleic acid sequencing offer the most sensitive ways to detect the viral genome in the clinical samples.

Different diagnosis : The disease should be differentiated from the following diseases.

(a) Foot and mouth disease : This is a highly infectious and contagious disease and spread by direct contact while bluetongue is not transmitted by direct contract but require insect vector for its transmission. FMD produces vesicles on the tongue and feet but there is no bluish coloration of the tongue. In bluetongue a pink line appears on coronet which is not present in foot and

mouth disease. In FMD there is no development of pulmonary oedema and pneumonia which is present in bluetongue disease.

(b) Malignant catarrhal fever (MCF) : There is extensive erosions on the buccal cavity, tongue, hard palate and fore stomachs but in bluetongue the lesions are not extensive in nature. MCF is sporadic in nature whereas bluetongue is seasonal in nature. Corneal opacity due to severe panopthalmitis is found in MCF but not in bluetongue.

(c) Photosensitization : There is dermatitis of light skin on exposure to light and is not caused by infection. In photosensitization there is reddening and oedema whereas in bluetongue there is erosion, oedema , necrosis and crust formation. Cyanosis of tongue mucosa and pink line in coronary band characteristic features of bluetongue are absent in photosensitization.

Treatment : There is no treatment against bluetongue. Antibiotic may be given through parenteral route to check secondary bacterial infection. Localized lesions may be treated with topical antiseptic solution or antibiotic powder to accelerate rate of healing. Affected animals should be kept away from solar exposure.

Control : The following measures may be undertaken to prevent and control the bluetongue.

1. Grazing of the animals should be avoided in areas where there is lot of culicoides vectors.
2. Attempts should be made to curb down the vector population by spraying insecticides and good water management.
3. Good hygienic and sanitary conditions should be adopted to control the spread of the disease.
4. Movement of all the animals susceptible to bluetongue should be restricted.
5. Contact with wild ruminants should be avoided.
6. Strict quarantine of the affected and sick animals should be made.
7. Animals importation from bluetongue disease prone countries should be strictly avoided.
8. Immunoprophylactic measures : In India there is no vaccine available which is effective against BT. However, in foreign countries both live attenuated and inactivated vaccines are available and routinely used to control the BT. In India, preliminary studies on the development and evaluation of inactivated (BEI, BPL and hydroxylamine) and adjuvanted (Aluminium hydroxide and saponin) BTV vaccines have shown the encouraging results in eliciting both humoral as well as cell mediated immunity in vaccinated animals which withstood challenge virus infection also.

Further reading

Boone, J.D., Balasuriya, U.B., Karaca, K., Audonnet, J.C., Yao, J. and He, L. (2007). Recombinant canarypox virus vaccine co-expressing genes encoding the VP2 and VP5 outer capsid proteins of bluetongue virus induces high level protection in sheep. *Vaccine* 25 (4): 672–8.

Boyce, M., Celma, C.C. and Roy, P. (2008). Development of reverse genetics systems for bluetongue virus: recovery of infectious virus from synthetic RNA transcripts. *J. Virol.* 82(17): 8339–48.

Celma, C.C. and Roy, P. (2009). A viral nonstructural protein regulates bluetongue virus trafficking and release. *J. Virol.* 83(13): 6806–16.

Clavijo, A., Heckert, R.A., Dulac, G.C. and Afshar, A.(2000). Isolation and identification of bluetongue virus. *J. Virol. Meth.* 87:13-23.

Dash, P.K., Nandi, S., Pande, A. and Mondal, B. and Bandyopadhyay, S.K. (2005). Comparative phylogenetic analysis of bluetongue virus based on sequencing of two different regions of L2 gene. *Indian J. Comp. Microbiol. Immunol. Infect. Dis.* 26: 2: 79-85.

Dash, P.K., Nandi, S., Pande, Amit., Mondal, B. and Bandyopadhyay, S.K. (2008). Molecular characterization of L2 gene of an Indian isolate of Bluetongue virus type-23. *Indian J. Virol.* 19(2): 183-190.

Elbers, A.R., Backx, A., Mintiens, K., Gerbier, G., Staubach, C. and Hendrickx, G. (2008). Field observations during the Bluetongue serotype 8 epidemic in 2006. II. Morbidity and mortality rate, case fatality and clinical recovery in sheep and cattle in the Netherlands. *Prev. Vet. Med.* 87 (1–2):31–40.

Hunter, P. and Modumo, J. (2001). A monovalent attenuated serotype 2 bluetongue virus vaccine confers homologous protection in sheep. *Onderstepoort J. Vet. Res.* 68(4):331–3.

Kumar, Pawan., Kumar, N., Kumar, P., Nandi, S. and Singh, V. (2008). Clinical and laboratory diagnosis of bluetongue viral disease. *Adv. Life Sci.* 1 : 3&4 : 92-96.

Lacetera, N. and Ronchi, B. (2004). Evaluation of antibody response and nonspecific lymphocyte blastogenesis following inoculation of a live attenuated bluetongue virus vaccine in goats. *Am. J. Vet. Res.* 65 (10):1331–4.

Lobato, Z.I., Coupar, B.E., Gray, C.P., Lunt, R. and Andrew, M.E. (1997). Antibody responses and protective immunity to recombinant vaccinia virus-expressed bluetongue virus antigens. *Vet. Immunol. Immunopathol.* 59 (3–4): 293–309.

Loudon, P.T., Hirasawa, T., Oldfield, S., Murphy, M. and Roy, P. (1991). Expression of the outer capsid proteinVP5 of two bluetongue viruses, and synthesis of chimeric double shelled virus-like particles using combinations of recombinant baculoviruses. *Virology.* 182 (2):793–801.

Mellor, P.S., Boorman, J. and Baylis, M. (2000). Culicoides biting midges: their role as arbovirus vectors. *Ann. Rev. Entomol.* 45: 307-340.

Mellor, P.S., Carpenter, S., Harrup, L., Baylis, M. and Mertens, P.P. (2008). Bluetongue in Europe and the Mediterranean Basin: history of occurrence prior to 2006. *Prev. Vet. Med.* 87(1–2): 4–20.

Murray, P.K. and Eaton, B.T.(1996).Vaccines for bluetongue. *Aus. Vet. J.* 73(6):207-10.

Nandi, S. (2006). Recent Developments in Bluetongue Vaccines. Lead paper presented in National Seminar on "Strategies for Control of Bluetongue", held at Deptt. Of Microbiology, CVS, Tirupati from May 24-25, 2006, pp 84-94.

Nandi, S., Pandey, A.B., Suresh, I. and Audarya, S.D. (2005). Seroprevalence of bluetongue disease in sheep by cELISA in Ahmedabad district of Gujarat state (India). *Indian J. Comp. Microbiol. Immunol. Infect. Dis.* 26: 1: 44-46.

Pandey, A.B., Nandi, S., Dwivedi, P. and Mehrotra, M.L. (2004). Bluetongue Disease. Technical bulletin published by CADRAD, IVRI, Izatnagar, U.P.

Ramakrishnan, M. A., Pandey, A. B., Singh, K. P., Singh, R., Nandi, S. and Mehrotra, M. L. (2006). Immunogenic responses and protective efficacy of BEI inactivated Bluetongue virus vaccines in sheep. *Veterinary Research Communications.* 30: 873-880.

Ramakrishnan, M. A., Singh, K. P., Pandey, A. B., Singh, R., Nandi, S. and Mehrotra, M. L. (2005). Genomic diversity of Indian isolates of bluetongue virus. *Acta Virologica.* 49: 285-286.

Roberts, D.H.(1990). Bluetongue: a review. *State Vet. J.* 44(124): 66-80.

Roy, P., Bishop, D.H., LeBlois, H. and Erasmus, B.J. (1994). Long-lasting protection of sheep against bluetongue challenge after vaccination with virus-like particles: evidence for homologous and partial heterologous protection. *Vaccine.* 12 (9): 805–11.

Roy, P., Boyce, M. and Noad, R. (2009). Prospects for improved bluetongue vaccines. *Nat. Rev.Microbiol.* 7(2):120–8.

Roy, P., French, T. and Erasmus, B.J. (1992). Protective efficacy of virus-like particles for bluetongue disease. *Vaccine.* 10(1): 28–32.

Roy, P., Urakawa, T., Van Dijk, A.A. and Erasmus, B.J. (1990). Recombinant virus vaccine for bluetongue disease in sheep. *J. Virol.* 64(5):1998–2003.

Savini, G., MacLachlan, N.J., Sanchez-Vizcaino, J.M., Zientara, S. (2008). Vaccines against bluetongue in Europe. *Comp. Immunol. Microbiol. Infect. Dis.* 31(2–3):101–20.

Sharifah, S.H., Ali, M.A., Gard, G.P. and Polkinghorne, I.G.(1995). Isolation of multiple serotypes of bluetongue virus from sentinel livestock in Malaysia. *Trop. Anim. Hlth. Prod.* 27(1): 37-42.

Shimshony, A., Barzilai, E., Savir, D. and Davidson, M.(1988). Epidemiology and control of bluetongue disease in Israel. *Rev. Sci. Tech. (OIE).* 7(2):311-329.

Singer, R.S., MacLachlan, N.J. and Carpenter, T.E.(2001). Maximal predicted duration of viremia in bluetongue virus-infected cattle. *J. Vet.Diag. Invest.* 13: 43-49.

Sreenivasulu, D., Rao, M.V.S. and Gard, G.P.(1999). Isolation of bluetongue virus serotype 2 from native sheep in India. *Vet. Rec.* 144(16): 452-453.

Vercauteren, G., Miry, C., Vandenbussche, F., Ducatelle, R., Van der Heyden, S. and Vandemeulebrouck E. (2008). Bluetongue virus serotype 8-associated congenital hydranencephaly in calves. *Transbound. Emerg. Dis.* 55(7):293–8.

Wade-Evans, A.M., Romero, C.H., Mellor, P., Takamatsu, H., Anderson, J. and Thevasagayam, J. (1996). Expression of the major core structural protein (VP7) of bluetongue virus, by a recombinant capripox virus, provides partial protection of sheep against a virulent heterotypic bluetongue virus challenge. *Virology.* 220(1): 227–31.

❑❑❑

8

Infectious Bovine Rhinotracheitis

Synonyms : Viral bovi. rhinotracheitis, Red nose, I.B.R, Infectious pustular vulvovaginits (IPV), Coital exanthema, Infectious pustular balanoposthitis (IPB), Bovine herpes virus 1(BHV 1).

It is a highly infectious disease of bovine characterized by high fever, rhinotracheitis, conjunctivitis, with a short course and high recovery rate. Encephalitis, the systemic form of the disease in new born calves, infectious pustular vulvovaginits/balanoposthitis are other syndromes caused by the same virus. Genetic isolates of various clinical isolates has found subtypes of BHV 1; a respiratory subtype BHV 1.1, a genital subtype BHV1.2 and an encephalatic subtype BHV 1.3, which is now termed as BHV 5.

Distribution : The disease is worldwide in distribution. The disease was first observed in USA in 1950. The name IPV has been assigned by Kendrik *et al.,* (1958). The disease has been identified in the USA, Australia, the U.K., Canada, New Zealand, South Africa and Zimbabwe and Europe.

Etiology : The disease is caused by bovid/bovine herpes virus 1 (BHV 1) under the subfamily *Alphaherpesviridae* and family *Herpesviridae.* It is an enveloped virus and about 150 nm in diameter. The ds DNA genome is wrapped around a fibrous spool like core, the fibers of which are anchored to the inner side of the surrounding capsid. The capsid is icosahedral in shape, 100 nm in diameter and composed of 162 hollow capsomers : 150 hexamers and 12 pentamers. There is a layer of globular material surrounding the capsid called tegument. It is enclosed by a typical lipoprotein envelope which carries the glycoprotein projections/spikes called peplomes. The virions are pleomorphic and diameter ranges from 120-200 nm.

The herpesvirus genome consists of a liner ds DNA molecule which is infectious under experimental condition. One unique feature of herpesvirus genome is the presence of high percentage of G+C percentage which varies from 32% (canine herpesvirus) to 74% (pseudorabies virus), a range exceeds percentage of G+C of all eukaryotes. The viruses under alphaherpesvirinae have the properties of affecting wide range of species, rapid growth and causing lysis of infected and establishing latent infections. The IBR virus causes different manifestations in cows (IPV) and bulls (IBP) indicating that virus with differing tissue affinities may exist in the field which can only be differentiated by immunological and biochemical means. There has been rare instances of respiratory and genital forms of the disease occurring together. It is also not possible to distinguish different field isolates from vaccine strain except deletion mutants. Using RE mapping of IBR virus isolates genome, it is possible to compare the antigenic differences between isolates obtained from different clinical syndromes and tissues.

Susceptible hosts : Cattle of all ages are susceptible to experimental challenge but the disease occurs naturally mostly in animals over 6 months of age. Dairy and beef cattle are equally susceptible. Alphaherpesvirus antigenically related to bovine herpesvirus 1 have been isolated from several ruminant species including red deer, rein deer, mule deer, pronghorn antelope, wildebeest etc. Buffalo and wildlife may play an important role in the maintenance of the infection. The disease can affect rarely swine naturally in both respiratory and genital form.

Mode of transmission : The main sources of infection are the nasal exudates and droplets, genital secretions, semen and fetal fluids and tissues. Aerosol is the important mode of transmission of respiratory disease ; veneral transmission is the method of spread of the genital disease. The IBR virus may survive for up to 1 year in semen frozen at -196°C. Introduction of new carrier/ infected animal may spread the disease.

One of the important features of the BHV-1 is its ability to become latent following primary infection with a mild strain or following vaccination with a live attenuated strain. The virus may remain latent indefinitely and recrudescence, reactivation and shedding of the virus may be possible by the use of large doses of corticosteroids which mimics the effects of stress. Animals vaccinated with attenuated strain can remain as carrier and vaccine strain does not provide protection against establishment of latent infection with a wild strain. Vaccination does not inhibit the excretion of wild strain which was latent at the time of vaccination.

Latency : The actual site of latency of BHV-1 is trigeminal ganglion. Calves may develop latency with virulent BHV-1 virus in trigeminal ganglion previously vaccinated with modified live vaccine. Recrudescence of the virus from the trigeminal ganglion and spread along the peripheral nerves by intra-axonal flow to the nasal mucosa can occur in calves under stress condition or treated with corticosteroids even in the presence of humoral antibodies. The virus has been recovered from the trigeminal ganglia of 10% of clinically normal cattle out of 40% which had serum neutralizing antibodies. This findings suggest that cattle from endemic herds must be considered as potential source of infection to other unexposed or healthy animals. Reactivation and shedding of the BHV-1 can occur in carrier bulls at the time of mating and virus has been detected in semen and preputial washing 2-3 months after last immunization with a live attenuated vaccine. However, the frequency of recurrent infection and shedding of virus has been reduced after vaccination. The reactivation and shedding of virus has been noticed in cows after parturition and in cattle after experimentally infected with *Dictyocaulus viviparous*. The placenta can harbour the virus during latent stage for up to 90 days without transmitting the virus to foetus.

The immunity to BHV-1 infection is complex and consists of both humoral and cell mediated immunity (CMI). The level of humoral immunity is an indicator of previous infection and an indirect measure of resistance to clinical disease. However, animals with low level of humoral antibodies may be immune to infection due to CMI. Local secretory antibody and interferon (IFN) are produced in animals following I/N infection or vaccination of live attenuated vaccine administered I/N. The IFN appears in 3 days and persists for 10 days. Animals are not immune to challenge infection 3 days after vaccination but by 7 days due to presence of antibodies in serum and nasal secretion. Calves acquire colostral antibodies which persist for 6 months and vaccination should be commenced when there is no maternal antibodies.

Pathogenesis : In the respiratory form of the disease , the virus multiplies in the nasal cavities and upper respiratory tract and causes rhinitis, laryngitis and tracheitis. There is extensive loss of cilia of trachea and pneumonia develops in severe infection. The virus is spread from nasal cavities to the ocular tissues through nasolacrymal duct and give rise to conjunctivitis, corneal oedema and deep vascularization. The virus may enter the brain tissues from nasal mucosa via trigeminal peripheral nerve to the trigeminal ganglion and produce non-suppurative meningoencephalitis. I/N inoculation of young calves and adult cows with BHV 1 can result in non-fatal trigeminal ganglionitis and encephaltitis which may be important mechanism of latent infection.

There is localization of the virus in several different tissues of animals following systemic invasion. The virus is transported by peripheral leukocytes to the placenta and foetus. Pregnant cows usually abort between the 5th and 9th month of pregnancy. Infection in the last trimester of gestation may result in mummification , abortion, still birth or weak calves. The systemic form of the disease in the new born calves is characterized by severe inflammatory and necrosis of respiratory and alimentary tract.

Cows develop acute necrotizing endometritis following I/U inoculation of the BHV-1. Focal necrosis and cellular infiltration in ovaries of heifer may be noticed in heifers following experimental inoculation of BHV1 during oestrus and insemination. Live attenuated vaccine strain of BHV 1 can produce similar lesions.

Clinical signs : The incubation period varies from 3-7 days following experimental infection and 10-20 days under natural condition.

The clinical signs may vary widely and have been grouped as :

- Respiratory form affecting respiratory tract.
- Genital form affecting genital tract.
- Ocular form affecting eyes.
- Encephalomyelitis form affecting CNS.
- Abortive form causing abortion.

Respiratory form : IBR occurs as a subclinical , mild or severe disease. Morbidity approaches 100% and mortality may reach 10%. This form is characterized by fever, inappetance, acceleration of respiration rate and dypsnoea. There is profuse nasal discharge, initially serous and later mucopurulent. The nasal mucosa is hyperemic and lesions progress from pustular necrosis to large haemorrhagic and ulcerated areas covered by a cream coloured diphtheric membrane. Foul breath, mouth breathing, salivation and a deep bronchial cough are common. The mortality rate is less unless there is secondary bacterial or viral infection. Animal may show signs of bronchitis and pneumonitis. The disease is called 'red nose' as there is red appearance of nasal mucosa. Acute uncomplicated cases last for 5-10 days and remain as carrier to shed virus for a considerable period.

Genital form : IPV is most commonly noticed in dairy cows. Affected animals develop fever, depression, anorexia and stand apart avoiding tail from contact with the vulva. Animals micturate at frequent intervals. Vulva may remain swollen and there may be mucopurulent discharge from vulva and vagina. Vestibular mucosa is reddened with many small pustules which coalesce to form fibrinous pseudomembrane that covers an ulcerated mucosa. The acute case of the disease lasts 4-5 days.

Occular form : There is inflammation of the conjunctiva (conjunctivitis) and serous to purulent ocular discharges. Petechial haemorrhages and corneal opacity may be evident. This form may appear along with respiratory form.

Encephalomyelitic form : The signs include high rise of temperature, incoordination, tremor, cycling, falling, coma and death of calves within 4 days from onset of neurological disorders.

Abortive form : There may be 'abortion storm' as cows may abort foetus died at 4 months of gestation. Foetus is autolysed and expelled within 1-7 days of death.

Lesions

System	Changes
Respiratory system	White necrotic foci are noted on the muzzle and nasal cavities. Lymph nodes in the throat and neck regions are usually swollen and oedematous. Due to considerable erosions of the nasal mucosa, the disease is called 'red nose'. Degenerative and necrotic changes are evident on the pharynx, larynx, trachea and terminate in the large bronchi. There may be pulmonary emphysema and secondary bronchopneumonia.
Reproductive system	Pustular lesion are noted on the mucosa of vulva and vagina. Foetus may undergo necrosis, mummification and autolysis. Necrotic lesions may appear in liver and spleen of the foetus.
Central nervous system	Lesions are noted on the cerebral cortex and the internal capsule. Cowdry type A inclusion bodies have been observed in the epithelial cells.

Diagnosis : Diagnosis is based on the clinical signs and characteristic lesions. The respiratory form of the disease may be confused with BVD, RP, MCF and pulmonary pasteurellosis. The nervous form may be confused with rabies and pseudorabies. The confirmatory diagnosis may be provided through laboratory tests e.g. virus isolation in MDBK cells and FAT using liver and spleen of the foetus. SNT is the routine serological test to evaluate antibody titre of current or recent infection. ELISA and dot-ELISA may provide alternative and sensitive method for diagnosis of the disease. Molecular biological techniques namely PCR, RE mapping, nucleic acid sequencing may be adopted for detection and characterization of viral genome/isolate.

Treatment : There is no treatment of the IBR. Secondary bacterial infection can be checked by broad spectrum antibiotics or sulphonamide. Treatment may be provided for fluid and electrolyte balance along with adequate ration and shelter may be provided. Hyperimmune serum may be tried but corticosteroid should not be given.

Control

1) Affected animals should be isolated from the healthy animals.
2) Number of live modified virus vaccines are available in some part of the world. In India, recently an inactivated IBR virus vaccine (IBRIVAX) grown in cell culture and emulsified with fortified special oil adjuvant has been introduced in the market by Intervet. Primary vaccination in young and adult animals should be carried out at 4-6 weeks of age and at any age respectively. All the animals should be given booster dose 3 months later followed by annual revaccination. The vaccine should be given @ 2 ml subcutaneously or intramuscularly.

Further Reading

Ackermann, M. and Wyler, R. (1984). The DNA of an IPV strain of bovid herpesvirus 1 in sacral ganglia during latency after intravaginal infection. *Vet. Microbiol.* 9 : 53-63.

Babiuk, L.A., van Drunen, Little-van den., Hurk, S. and Tikoo, S.K. (1996) Immunology of bovine herpesvirus 1 infection. *Vet. Microbiol.* 53 : 31-42.

Bitsch, V. (1973). Bovine rhinotracheitis virus infection in bulls, with special reference to preputial infection. *Appl. Microbiol.* 26 : 337-343.

Boelaert, F., Speybroeck, N., de Kruif, A., Burzykowski, T., Molenberghs, G. and Berkven, D.L. (2005). Risk factors for bovine herpesvirus -1 seropositivity. *Prev. Vet. Med.* 69: 3-4: 285-295.

Boelaert, F., Biront, P., Soumare, B., Dispas, M., Vanopdenbosch, E., Vermeersch, J.P., Raskin, A., Dufey, J., Berkvens, D. and Kerkhofs, P. (2000). Prevalence of bovine herpesvirus 1 in Belgian cattle population. *Prev. Vet. Med.* 45 : 285 -295.

Brake, F. and Studdert, M.J. (1985). Molecular epidemiology and pathogenesis of ruminant herpesviruses including bovine buffalo and caprine herpesviruses 1 and bovine encephalitis herpesvirus. *Aust. Vet. J.* 62 : 331-334.

Edwards, S., Newman, R.H. and White, H. (1991). The virulence of British isolates of BHV-1 in relationship to viral genotype. *British Vet. J.* 47 : 216-231.

Edwards, S., White, H. and Nixon, P. (1990). A study of the predominant genotypes of BHV-1 found in UK. *Vet. Microbiol.* 22: 213-223.

Frerichs, G.N., Woods, S.B., Lucas, M.H. and Sands, J.J. (1982). Safety and efficacy of live and inactivated infectious bovine rhinotracheitis vaccines. *Vet. Rec.* 111 : 116-122.

Fuchs, M., Hubert, P., Detterer, J. and Rziha, H.J. (1999). Detection of bovine herpesvirus type a1 in blood from naturally infected cattle by using a sensitive PCR that discriminates between wild type virus and virus lacking glycoprotein *Eur. J. Clin. Microbiol.* 37 : 2498-2507.

Galiero, G., Giordanelli, M.P. and Fraulo, P. (2001). Infectious bovine rhinotracheitis (IBR). Note 1 : serum epidemiological survey in buffalo herds of southern Italy. *Bubalus-Bubalis.* 7(4) : 69-74.

Gibbs, E.P.J. and Rweyemamu, M.M. (1977). Bovine herpesviruses. Part I. Bovine herpesvirus 1. *Vet. Bull.* 47 : 317-

Leite, F., Sylte, M.J., O'Brien, S., Schultz, R., Peek, S., van Reeth, K. and Czuprynski, C.J. (2002). Effect of experimental infection of cattle with bovine herpesvirus1 (BHV-1) on the *ex vivo* interaction of bovine leukocytes with *Mannheimia (Pasteurella) haemolytica* leukotoxin. *Vet.Immunol. Immunopathol.* 84 :97-100.

Metzler, A.E., Matile, H., Gassmann, U., Engels, M. and Wyler, R. (1985). European isolates of BHV-1 : a comparison of RE sites, polypeptides and reactivity with monoclonal antibodies. *Arch. Virol.* 85: 57-69.

Miller, J.M., Whetstone, C.A. and Van der Maarten, M.J. (1991). Abortifacient property of BHV-1 isolates that represent three subtypes of determined by RE analysis of viral DNA. *Amer. J. Vet. Res.* 52: 458-461.

Msolla, P.M., Allan, E.M., Selman, J.E. and Wiseman, A. (1983). Reactivation and shedding of bovine herpesvirus 1 following *Dictyocaulus viviparous* infection. *J. Comp. Path.* 93 : 271-274.

Murphy, F.A., Gibbs, E.P.J., Horzinek, M.C. and Studdert, M.J. (1999). Veterinary Virology, Third Ed, Academic Press, New York.

Noordegraaf, A.V., Jalvingh, A.W., de Jong, M.C.M., Franken, P. and Dijkhuizen, A.A. (2000). Evaluating control strategies for outbreaks in BHV-1 free areas including stochastic and spatial simulation. *Prev. Vet. Med.* 44: 21-42.

Parsonson, I.M. and Snowdon, W.A. (1975). The effect of natural and artificial breeding using bulls infected with or semen contaminated with infectious bovine rhinotracheitis virus. *Australian Vet. J.* 51 : 365-369.

Pastoret, P.P., Thiry, E., Brochier, B. and Derboven, G. (1982). Bovine herpesvirus 1 infection of cattle : pathogenesis, latency, consequences of latency. *Ann. Res. Vet.* 13 : 221-235.

Rocha, M.A., Barbosa, E.F., Guimaraes, S.E.F., Dias, N. E. and Gomcia, A.M.G. (1998). A high sensitivity-nested PCR assay for BHV-1 detection in semen of naturally infected bulls. *Vet. Microbiol.* 63 : 1-11.

Rossi, C.R., Kiesel, G.K. and Rumph, P.F.(1982). Association between route of inoculation with infectious bovine rhinotracheitis virus and site of recrudescence after dexamethasone treatment. *Amer. J. Vet. Res.* 43 : 1440-1442.

Salwa, A., Rulka, J. and Arent, Z.(2000). The prevalence of the mixed infection of BLV, BHV-1, BVD-MD in dairy herds. *Medycina Weterynaryjna.* 56 (7) : 443-444.

Schudel, A.A., Carillo, B.J., Wyler, R. and Metzler, A.E. (1986). Infections of calves with antigenic variants of BHV 1 and neurological disease. *J.Vet.Med.* 33B : 303-310.

Schultz, R.D., Hall, C.E., Sheffy, B.E., Kahrs, R.F. and Bean, B.H. (1977). Current status of IBR-IPV infection in bulls. In : Proc. 80th Ann. Meeting. US Anim. Health Ass. 159-168.

Straub, O.C. (1990). IBR virus In : Virus infections of ruminants (Z Dinter and B Morein Eds) Elsevier Science Publishers BV, Oxford.

Turin, L. and Russo, S. (2003). BHV-1 infection in cattle : an update. *Vet. Bull.*73:16R-21R.

Van Oirschot, J.T. (1995). Bovine herpesvirus 1 in semen of bulls and the risk of transmission : a brief review. *Vet. Quart.* 17: 29-33.

Wentink, G.H., Rutten, V.P.M.G., van Exsel, A.C.A., de Jong, W.A.C., Vleugel, H. and Hensen, E.J. (1990). Failure of an in vitro lymphoproliferative assay specific for bovine herpes virus type 1 to detect immunized or latently infected animals. *Vet. Quart.* 12 : 175-182.

Wentink, G.H., van Oirschot, J.T. and Verhoeff, J. (1993). Risk of infection with BHV-1 : a review. *Vet. Quart.* 15: 30-33.

White, M.B. and Snowdon, W.A. (1973). The breeding record of cows inseminated with a batch of semen contaminated with infectious bovine rhinotracheitis virus. *Aust. Vet. J.* 49 : 501-506.

Winkler, M.T.C., Doster, A. and Jones, C. (1999) Bovine herpesvirus 1 can infect CD4+ T lymphocytes and induce programmed cell death during acute infection of cattle. *J. Virol.* 73 : 8657-8668.

Winkler, M.T.C., Doster, A. and Jones, C. (2000) Persistence and reactivation of bovine herpesvirus 1 in the tonsils of latently infected calves. *J. Virol.* 74 : 5337-5346.

Zhou, J., Lyaku, J., Fredrickson, R.A. and Kibenge, F.S.B. (1999). Improved detection of bovine herpesvirus 1 in artificially infected bovine semen by protein amplification. *J. Virol. Meth.* 79 : 181-189.

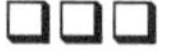

9

Bovine Ephemeral Fever

Synonyms : Three days sickness, Stiff sickness, Dengu fever of cattle, Bovine epizootic fever and Lazy man's disease.

Bovine ephemeral fever (BEF) is a viral disease of cattle, *Bos Taurus*, *Bos indicus* and *Bos javanicus* and water buffalo *Bubalus bubalis*, although subclinically infect a greater range of ruminant species. Although the disease has a variety of names, bovine ephemeral fever is most commonly used and is very apt. The disease in cattle is characterized by acute febrile reaction, stiffness, lameness and spontaneous recovery in three days. The morbidity may be high but the mortality is low. It mainly occurs in subtropical and temperate regions of Africa, Asia and Australia.

Distribution : The origin of ephemeral fever is obscure. The first reports of the ephemeral fever were probably in mid-nineteenth century when the disease was first noticed in East Africa and subsequently in Rhodesia, Kenya, South Africa, Indonesia, India, Egypt, Palestine, Australia and in 1949 in Japan. The disease may be epidemic in much of Africa and Southern Asia since antiquity but the disease has spread to a wide area due to development of more intensive cattle industry. The disease is prevalent in tropical, subtropical and some temperate regions of Africa, Australia and Asia. The disease has never been reported in Western hemisphere, North and South America. New Zealand and Pacific Islands are free from the disease. In South Africa, India, Japan and parts of Australia the disease is enzootic.

Etiology : Bovine ephemeral fever is caused by BEF virus, a single stranded negative sense RNA virus under the genus *Ephemerovirus* and family *Rhabdoviridae.* The virus is bullet shaped, enveloped and measures 80X120-140 nm with a fringe of fine surface projections. Although most of the BEF virus are bullet shaped, south African strains are mostly conical but closely related to bullet shaped Asian and Australian strains serologically. There are four serotypes of BEF virus namely DDP63, CSIRO 368, DDP61 and FUK 11. As the BEF virus is enveloped, it is sensitive to diethylether and sodium deoxycholate. Citrated whole blood from BEF affected animals remain infective at 4°C. There is loss of infectivity of BEF virus at low pH (2.5) or high pH (12.0) within 10 minutes. The virus is inactivated within 10 minutes at 56°C and 18 hours at 37°C.

Susceptible hosts : Both indigenous and exotic breeds of cattle as well as water buffalo are susceptible. Although all age groups are susceptible, the disease is more common in adults. However, calves are equally susceptible to adults following experimental infection. Newborn colostrums deprived calves are susceptible. Water buffaloes are susceptible to ephemeral fever but in Australia they are refractory to experimental infection. Subclinical infection in Australian water buffalo is common as judged by serological studies. The role of wildlife as reservoir host is still obscure. In Kenya, the antibody to BEF virus has been demonstrated in African buffalo, water buck, wildebeest and hartebeest. Domestic and feral red deer in Australia have a high prevalence of neutralizing antibody. Sheep and other domestic animals are not susceptible, though passaging of BEF virus through sheep experimentally has become possible. Repeated I/C passages in suckling mice produces strains pathogenic for adult mice by I/C inoculation. Adult rats, guinea pigs and lambs are susceptible.

Mode of transmission : The disease is transmitted by sand fly (Ceratopogonidae family). In recent years, mosquitoes like *Culex sp.*, *Anopheles sp.* and *Aedes sp.* have been suggested as disease transmitter. Transmission does not occur by direct contact with infected animals or their saliva or ocular discharges. The disease is not transmitted through semen. Bovine ephemeral fever is most prevalent during rainy seasons when the insects are numerous and the spread is influenced by the wind movement. The virus is associated with the leucocytes fractions of blood and the disease is easily transmitted by inoculating I/V blood taken from diseased animals showing febrile reactions to susceptible cattle. Mechanical transmission through insect or by direct contact does not occur and the virus does not persist 4th day after the subsidence of fever. Animals once infected confer lifelong immunity although second time attack two to three weeks apart is not uncommon.

Pathogenesis : The pathogenesis is complex and the release of lymphokines mediates the host inflammatory process resulting the final outcome of the disease. The incubation period is usually 2 to 10 days. The virus multiplies in the blood followed by localization in the mesodermal tissues like joints, muscle, lymph nodes and thereby clinical manifestation like dyspnoea, limb stiffness develop. The virus multiplies in the reticuloendothelial cells, in the lungs, spleen, lymph nodes rather than lymphoid cells or vascular endothelium. In every case there is early neutrophilia with an abnormal level of immature neutrophil in the circulation. There is significant drop in plasma calcium and elevated level of plasma fibrinogen. Affected animals respond well to non-steroid anti-inflammatory agents and calcium infusion. There is solid immunity in animals following infection and repeat clinical episode usually involve the newborn or young calves.

Clinical signs : BEF virus infection of cattle can be expressed in different forms from imperceptible clinical signs to death. The host response to infection and the environment heavily influence the severity and final outcome of the disease. The disease is more severe in adult cattle than in young animal ; in fat animals than in lean animals, in heavy bulls than in light steers, in high lactating cattle than in dry cows. If affected cattle are without shade and water, they may suffer from severe dehydration.

The natural case of BEF is characterized by sudden onset of fever (41-42°C), lameness along with listlessness, inappetence and a starring coat followed by lachrymation, serous oral and nasal discharges, joint pain and general stiffness. The fever in BEF is biphasic, triphasic or occasionally multiphasic. The first phase body temperature is always lower than in later phase. Rumianal function may cease resulting in constipation. Lactation may decline suddenly or completely in dairy cows. In most of the cases, milk production returns normal progressively with recovery but level is always lower than preillness. In most of the cases there is temporary or permanent paralysis of all the forelegs. The paralysed cattle maintain sternal recumbency but in later stage they assume lateral recumbency. There is salivation and difficulty in swallowing. Bloat is a variable phenomenon. There is progressive loss of reflexes, coma and death occurs within 1-4 days after paralysis. Complete recovery occurs in 95-97% cases irrespective of mild or severe nature of clinical signs.

Complications usually occur and are manifested by pneumonia, mastitis, hind quarter paralysis, abnormal gait, abortion in late pregnancy and temporary infertility in bulls (up to 6 months). Pulmonary and subcutaneous emphysema are rare. All the changes are not observed in one outbreak. Climatic condition determined the severity of the clinical signs. Dairy cows in early and mid lactation are more likely to die than dry cows.

Pathology : BEF is an inflammatory disease, serofibrinous polysinovitis, polyarthritis, polytendovaginitis, cellulitis and focal necrosis of skeletal muscles are the common pathological lesions. There is enlargement and oedema of the lymph nodes. Lungs and pleura may show congestion and fatty oedema. Oedema and haemorrhages of the brain and meninges are noted.

Microscopically, there is neutrophilia, leucocytosis and high fibrogen level. A steady reduction in erythrocyte number initially followed by a larger fall which corresponded to haemosiderosis of lymph node and spleen. Lesions have been described in venules and capillaries in tendon sheath, synovial membranes, muscle, fascia and endothelium, perivascular neutrophilic infiltration, focal or complete necrosis of vessel walls, thrombosis and perivascular fibrosis.

Diagnosis : Ephemeral fever is usually diagnosed from history and clinical signs. A diagnosis can be made from the sudden onset of febrile reactions lasting for 2-5 days with spontaneous recovery. The seasonal occurrence and symptoms of oropharyngeal secretions, joint pain and stiffness are characteristics of BEF virus infections. However, a confirmatory diagnosis can be obtained by isolation of BEF virus from blood taken into heparin or EDTA anti-coagulant during fever or by demonstration of neutralizing and complement fixing antibodies in paired sera collected during illness and two or three weeks later. Fluorescent antibody test can be carried out to detect viral antigen in the cytoplasm of the leucocytes made from the smears of infected blood. The virus can also be isolated by inoculating blood from clinically cattle to susceptible or unweaned mice. Serological diagnosis can be complicated by the previous infection of antigenically related virus such as Kimberley virus. Kimberley virus infection is subclinical and causes the development of low titre of serum neutralizing antibodies to BEF virus without conferring any protection against BEF virus. A prior infection Kimberley virus sensitizes the cattle so that a secondary instead of primary antibody response occurs on first exposure to BEF virus. Kotonkan virus injected to cattle can produce clinical signs similar to BEF.

Differential diagnosis : The disease may be confused with milk fever or laminitis. Laminitis is local problem of the concerned foot and milk fever goes through 3 distinct stages viz., excitement stage, sternal recumbency stage and stage of lateral recumbency and paresis. Milk fever responds well with calcium therapy.

Treatment : Rational treatment will be of very effective if applied early in BEF cases. First, the affected cattle should be provided complete rest during acute illness and convalescence. Second, symptomatic treatment with anti-inflammatory drug viz., salicylates or phenylbutazone have been found to be beneficial. A variety of antibiotics can be used to check the secondary bacterial infections. The I/V or S/C administration of calcium borogluconate has been found to be beneficial to some but not all cattle. Isotonic fluids have been used to restore dehydration. During acute stage, no medicine should be given orally to avoid inhalation pneumonia due to inability of the animal to swallow.

Control : As it is a vector borne disease, control of vector is the important key to curb down the disease propagation. A variety of vaccines have been tried from time to time with inconsistent results. At present no vaccine is available in India. A single attack of BEF virus confers lifelong immunity to cattle. A killed vaccine can provide 6 months protection against BEF or be administered as an booster dose to cattle previously given live attenuated BEF virus vaccine. Attempts have been made to develop live attenuated vaccines by passaging the virus in mice or cell culture system. But loss of immunogenicity and virulence with increase of the passage level has become an impeding factor in the development of vaccine. The adjuvants which are used to enhance the antigenicity of live attenuated vaccines are Freund's incomplete adjuvant (south Africa), aluminium hydroxide and Quil A (Australia). In Japan, aluminium phosphate gel is used with the killed vaccine but not with the live vaccine.

Future reading

Abu Elzein, E.M.E., Gameel, A.A. and Al-Afaleq, A.I. (1999). Observations on the recent epizootic of bovine ephemeral fever in Saudi Arabia. *Rev. Sci. Tech.* 18(3): 672–680.

Abu Elzein, E.M.E., Gameel, A.A., Al Afaleq, A.I., Al Gundi, O. and Bukhari, A. (1997). Bovine ephemeral fever in Saudi Arabia. *Vet. Rec.* 140(24): 630–631.

Al-Busaidy, S.M. and Mellor, P.S. (1991). Isolation and identification of arboviruses from the Sultanate of Oman. *Epid. Infect.* 106(2): 403–413.

Braverman, Y. and Chechik, F. (1996). Air streams and the introduction of animal diseases borne on *Culicoides* (Diptera, Ceratopogonidae) into Israel. *Rev. Sci. Tech.* 15(3):1037–1052.

Burgess, G.W. (1971). Bovine ephemeral fever: a review. *Vet. Bull.* 141: 887–895.

Farag, M.A., Al-Sukayran, A., Mazloum, K.S. and Al-Bukomy, A.M. (1998). Epizootics of bovine ephemeral fever on dairy farms in Saudi Arabia. *Rev. Sci. Tech.* 17(3): 713–722.

Kirkland, P.D. (2002). Akabane and bovine ephemeral fever virus infections. *Vet. Clin. North Am. Food Anim. Pract.* 18: 501-14.

Murray, M.D. (1997). Possible vectors of bovine ephemeral fever in the 1967/68 epizootic in northern Victoria. *Aust. Vet. J.* 75(3): p. 220.

Nandi, S. and Negi, B.S. (1999). Bovine ephemeral fever: a review. *Comp. Immunol. Microbiol. Infect. Dis.* 22: 81–91.

St George, T.D. (1988). Bovine ephemeral fever: a review. *Trop. Anim. Hlth. Prod.* 120(4):194–202.

Stram, Y., Kuznetzova, L., Levin, A., Yadin, H. and Rubinstein-Giuni, M. (2005). A real-time RT-quantative (q)PCR for the detection of bovine ephemeral fever virus. *J. Virol . Meth.* 130: 1-6.

Uren, M.F., St. George, T.D. and Murphy, G.M. (1992). Studies on the pathogenesis of bovine ephemeral fever in experimental cattle III. Virological and biochemical data. *Vet. Microbiol.* 30(4): 297–307.

Uren, M.F., St George, T.D., Kirkland, P.D., Stranger, R.S. and Murray, M.D. (1987). Epidemiology of bovine ephemeral fever in Australia 1981–1985. *Aust. J. Biol. Sci.* 40(2):125–136.

Venter, G.J., Hamblin, C. and Paweska, J.T. (2003). Determination of the oral susceptibility of South African livestock-associated biting midges, *Culicoides* species, to bovine ephemeral fever virus. *Med. Vet. Entomol.* 17(2):133–137.

Walker, P.J. (2005). Bovine ephemeral fever in Australia and the world. *Curr. Top. Microbiol. Immunol.* 292: 57-80.

Wenbin, B., Chunling, J. and Davis, S.S. (1991). Preliminary observations on the epidemiology of bovine ephemeral fever in China. *Trop. Anim. Hlth Prod.*23(1): 22–26.

Yeruham, I., Braverman, Y. and Yadin, H. (2002). Epidemiological investigations of outbreaks of bovine ephemeral fever in Israel. *Vet. Rec.* 151(4):117–121.

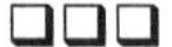

10

Canine Parvovirus Infections in Dog

Canine parvovirus 2 (CPV-2), the causative agent of acute haemorrhagic enteritis and myocarditis in dogs, is one of the most important pathogenic viruses. It is a highly contagious and often fatal disease. CPV-2 was first recognized in 1977 and since then it has been well established as an enteric pathogen of dogs throughout the world causing high morbidity (100%) and frequent mortality up to 10%. The disease is characterized by 2 prominent clinical forms (i) enteritis with vomition and diarrhea in dogs of all ages (ii) myocarditis and subsequent heart failure in pups of less than 3 months of age. The virus was named CPV-2 in order to differentiate it from a closely related parvovirus of canine known as CPV-1 or minute virus of canine (MVC). MVC, a completely different parvovirus, had not been associated with natural disease until 1992. MVC may cause pneumonia, myocarditis and enteritis in young pups or transplacental infections in pregnant dams, with embryo resorptions and fetal death. About 30 confirmed cases of CPV-1 have been reported in USA, Sweden, Germany and more recently in Italy. The canine parvovirus infections have been confined to be a problem in dogs in spite of a number of potent and efficacious live as well as inactivated vaccines available to be used in the dogs. So, it is the prime time to create awareness among the dog owners, pet lovers, Kennel club owners, pet shop owners and defense personnel about the disease in order to prevent and control the disease in a more effective and efficient manner.

Etiology : CPV is extremely small, 22 nm in diameter with an icosahedral capsid enclosing a genome composed of single stranded negative sense DNA of about 5.2 Kb in length coding two structural proteins (VP1 and VP2) and two non-structural proteins (NS1 and NS2). The CPV-2 is closely related antigenically to feline panleukopenia virus (FPLV) and appears to have arisen as a result of mutation of feline virus. The virus lacks envelope and essential lipid. Simply, one million virus particles laid end to end would measure slightly under one inch. There are a total of 60 copies of the VP1 and VP2 with about 5-6 copies of VP1 and 54-55 copies of VP2. Like all other parvoviruses, it can replicate only in actively dividing cells.

The virus can be grown in both primary dog kidney and cat kidney and CRFK, MDCK and A72 cell lines. But the growth in cell culture is not generally accompanied by a gross cytopathic effect although I/N inclusions may be found on microscopic examination. The presence of virus is normally detected by haemagglutinination, immunofluorescence, IPT or ELISA. Viral haemagglutination is also easily detected in the faeces of dogs with parvovirus enteritis.

As the virus is naked , it is resistant to ether and chloroform and stable at pH 3 and 9. The virus can withstand high temperature and can remain viable in fomites for many years. The virus is destroyed by 2% formalin, 2% NaOH and 2% sodium hypochloride. A typical average infectious dose for an unvaccinated dog is 1000 virus particles and chances of getting infections depend on the breed, age, health status of the dogs and virulence of the virus. An infected dog sheds 35 million viral particles (35000 times the typical infectious dose) per ounce of stool.

Antigenic variants of CPV-2 : Since the emergence of CPV-2 in 1978, an antigenic variant was identified in 1979 in many different countries of the world using monoclonal antibody testing and that strain was termed as CPV-2a. Although those viruses differed only in 5-6 amino acids from the CPV-2, they differed in two different neutralizing antigenic sites on the surface of the capsid. In 1984, a further antigenically variant virus strain was detected which differed in only a single epitope compared to CPV-2a and designated as CPV-2b. The only significant difference between CPV-2a and CPV-2b variants is the substitution of one amino acid (Asn to Asp) at position 426 of VP2 protein. Despite the small number of differences between these viruses in each case the viruses became globally distributed indicating that they must have been under strong selection. These viruses also differ in host range as well as antigenicity. The different antigenic variants of CPV are prevalent in varying proportion in different countries with >80% of isolates being CPV-2b and <20% CPV-2a in USA, while 60% are CPV-2a and 40% CPV-2b in Germany. In India, large number of positive cases of CPV infections are detected in samples of dogs collected from the Polyclinic, IVRI, or samples of dogs received from BSF, Tekanpur, Gwalior and Veterinary Polyclinic, Durg, Chhattisgarh on the basis of the results revealed in PCR. Besides, the disease has been reported by various workers viz., G.B. Pant University of Agriculture and Technology, Pantnagar, Uttarakhand, Punjab Agriculture University, Ludhiana, Veterinary College, Parbhani and Veterinary College, Madras etc on the basis of HA test, ELISA, LAT or PCR. From this study, the gravity of problem can be easily realized and suitable measures must be undertaken immediately to check the spread of the disease in the form of effective and efficient preventive and control programmes against the disease.

Host range : All the members of the group comprising CPV/FPLV replicate in feline cells in tissue culture, but only isolates from dogs replicate in cultured canine cells. Their *in vivo* host ranges also differ since FPLV isolates replicate efficiently only in cats whereas CPV isolate show variable replication in cats depending on the strain of CPV. The original CPV-2 isolates do not replicate in cats but the variants of CPV-2 designated CPV2a and CPV-2b replicate efficiently in cats.

Pathogenesis : CPV-2 replicates in several lymphoid tissues and the intestinal epithelium of dogs and FPLV replicates in the corresponding tissues in the cat. However, there are differences in the extent of viral growth in tissues of the two species. The pathogenesis of CPV-2 infections in dogs and FPLV infections in cats are very similar. The route of entry and initial site of virus replication are cells of nasal and oropharynx including tonsils and other lymphoid tissues. Animals can be experimentally infected by most of the parenteral routes but oral route is the most common natural route of infection. During viraemia, virus spread systematically and is found in tonsils, retropharyngeal lymph nodes, thymus and mesenteric lymph node after 1-3 days. The virus can be recovered by 3rd day in the Peyer's patches. Cytokines may play an important role in the pathogenesis of CPV/FPLV infections.

In general FPLV replicate in feline tissues, lymph node, thymus, spleen, intestinal epithelial cells and virus is present in large numbers in stools. It also replicates in thymus and bone marrow of dog but not in gut or mesenteric lymph node and there is no shedding of virus in the stool On the other hand, CPV-2, 2a and 2b have the ability to infect the gut tissues of dogs and virus is present in huge quantity in the stool. However, CPV-2 does not replicate in cats but CPV-2a and CPV-2b replicate in cats and high titre virus is present in lymphoid and intestinal tissue.

Epidemiology : In 1978, the entire canine populations was susceptible to CPV-2. Consequently, the infection and disease occurred in all ages of dogs from neonate pups to aged animals. The disease was first noticed predominantly in Kennels and both myocardial and enteric forms were seen.

Epidemiology is concerned with the frequency and distribution of diseases in populations. The pattern of disease experienced in a population is largely influenced by the susceptibility of the host, environmental and management conditions such as housing, hygiene and population density and pathogenicity of the infectious agent. The virus is present in high titers in the faeces of dogs during the acute phase of the disease and the faeces may remain infectious to other dogs for several weeks following clinical recovery. CPV-2 is transmitted from dog to dog primarily by faecal oral route. The constant introduction of susceptible pups (e.g. kennels) or import (pet shops) and improper environmental sanitation makes the dogs exposed to CPV-2 constantly.

Since CPV-2 virus excreted in the faeces is extremely resistant to inactivation and persists in the environment for prolonged periods of time, CPV-2 infection typically occurs in pups from weaning to about 20 weeks of age at a low but constant rate. However, due to interruptions in the vaccination programme or lapses in hygiene, outbreaks of CPV-2 enteritis associated with high rates of morbidity and mortality are common. All the vaccinated dogs in a Kennel will be naturally infected with CPV-2 when their maternal antibody titer declines below a critical level, although all infected dogs will not necessarily develop clinical disease. Adult dogs in kennel and pet shops are usually immune to CPV-2 infection either as a result of previous vaccination or natural exposures.

The differences in exposure patterns to CPV-2 between kennel dogs and household pups partially explains why CPV-2 vaccination has been very effective in reducing the incidence of CPV-2 enteritis in the pet dog populations. The annual number of cases and death due to CPV-2 in pet dogs has drastically reduced. Routine use of modified live CPV-2 vaccines for pups has resulted in a dramatic decrease in the incidence of CPV-2 enteritis in pet dogs. In contrast, outbreaks of CPV-2 enteritis continue to be a problem in kennel, pet shops and street dog populations. CPV-2 associated myocarditis resulting from infection of neonatal pups born to CPV-2 naïve dams has virtually disappeared as a clinical entity, because virtually all dams are now immune to the disease and passively transfer protective maternal antibodies through colostrum to the offspring.

Clinical signs : Two forms of clinical manifestations are observed in parvovirus infections (a) Parvovirus enteritis (b) Parvovirus myocarditis.

(a) Parvovirus enteritis : This occurs in dogs of any age but appears in serious proportions in pups. The most commonly encountered clinical signs include in order of decreasing frequency depression , vomition, diarrhea , anorexia and fever. There is slight rise of temperature in the initial stage of the disease but gradually turn to subnormal level with advancement of vomition and diarrhea. There is no consistent character of the stool, it may be watery, yellow in color or tinged with frank blood. The course of illness is also highly variable depending on the infectious dose of the virus and clinical signs usually develop from 3 days following infection and typically persist for 5 to 7 days. The morbidity and mortality vary according to the age of the animals, the severity of challenge and the presence of intercurrent disease problems. Faeces can vary from simply soft or pasty in mild cases to grossly haemmorhagic in severe cases. Death ensues due to dehydration leading to the peripheral circulatory failure.

It is important to realize that within a group of dogs or litter of dogs, there may be one death, two pups seriously ill, two pups slightly ill and 3 apparently unaffected. All however will excrete the virus in the faeces and develop a high antibody titer to the virus.

(b) Parvovirus myocarditis : CPV-2 myocarditis is a condition of young dogs (less than 10 weeks) and outstandingly a litter problem. Within an infected litter, 70% pups will die due to heart failure by 8 weeks of age and the remaining 30% will have pathological changes which may result in death many months or even years later. The most dramatic manifestations of CPV-2 myocarditis is the sudden death in young pups usually about 4 weeks of age. The collapsed dying pup may have cold extremities, pale mucosae and show gasping respiration or terminal convulsions. Acute heart failure with respiratory distress occurs in pups between 4 to 8 weeks of age. Subacute heart failure occurs in older pups usually 8 weeks or more. They are tachypnoeic or dyspnoeic especially on exercise. The abdomen is swollen with hepatomegaly and ascitic fluid is blood tinged. There is tachycardia, sometimes with arrhythmias and a weak pulse. Most animals die due to cardiogenic shock. However, if the animal survives it will suffer from chronic myocardial and circulatory complications. In pregnant bitches infection with CPV may cause lesions in placenta and infect foetus and lead to abnormality like cerebellar hypoplasia with little or no clinical findings in bitches.

Pathology : The pathological changes produced by CPV reflect the requirement of virus for dividing cells. The mesenteric and peripheral lymph nodes are enlarged and oedematous soon after infection and later may decrease in size. The thymus undergoes atrophy and can be reduced to $1/3^{rd}$ of the original size. There is extensive lysis of lymphocytes in all lymphoid tissues resulting in lymphocyte depletion. Lymphocytolysis is more severe in the cortex than in the medulla of the thymus. In other tissues, germinal centres are severely affected. There may be erythrocytic, myeloid and megakaryocytic cells in the bone marrow. Intranuclear (I/N) inclusion are rarely seen in the lymphoid tissue. Varying degree of immunosuppression is observed in CPV-2 infected dogs due to pathogenic changes in the lymphoid tissues.

The serosa of the small intestine is often haemorrhagic and has a fine granular appearance due to fibrinous effusion. The intestinal contents may be mucoid or haemorrhagic. The microscopic lesions vary from villus atrophy and crypt cell necrosis to severe loss of enterocytes. Later, there is epithelial regeneration characterized by presence of cuboidal or large irregularly shaped enterocytes and crypt cell hyperplasia. There is infiltration of neutrophils and eosinophils in the mucosa. Eosinophilic I/N inclusions are occasionally observed in intact crypt cells.

Post mortem examination of pups with myocarditis which die suddenly or due to acute heart failure may reveal severe pulmonary oedema with frothy fluid in the tracheobronchial tree. Microscopically, I/N basophilic inclusion bodies are commonly present in cardiac myocytes in the early stages and EM shows parvovirus particles in these nuclei.

In older animals (usually 8 weeks or older) with subacute heart failure, there is pulmonary oedema, hydrothorax, hydropericardium and ascites with hepatic enlargement and congestion. The heart is enlarged and dilated with pale streaks in the heart wall. Histologically, lymphoid tissues in myocarditis cases show reactive hyperplasia rather than lymphocytolysis.

Diagnosis : A presumptive diagnosis of CPV-2 enteritis can be made based on the age of the dog (<24 weeks of age), a history of inadequate vaccination for CPV-2 and clinical signs. Several laboratory tests have been developed and are available for specific viral diagnosis. Rapid diagnosis can be made by electron microscopy of faecal material from cases with typical signs of diseases. The virus also can be isolated in several feline and canine cell lines such as MDCK, CRFK and A-72 cell lines. But isolation is seldom practised since cell culture requires at least 1 week to provide diagnosis. Faecal HA and HI test have provided a simple and rapid method for detecting virus in faecal and tissue samples and are adopted by several diagnostic laboratories. However, the HA test is less sensitive than EM or ELISA. Several species of RBC e.g. pig, rhesus monkey or cat can be used to perform the test. For specificity, a HI test is needed to be carried out using specific antiserum or MAbs. (The rapid antigen test kits are available in India and abroad to dingnose the CPV disease.) This test is based on the antigen-antibody reactions with specific MAbs fixed on plastic, nitrocellulose membranes, latex or gold particles. The tests are rapid, relatively cheap and can be performed in any veterinary clinic.

Recently, polymerase chain reaction has been adopted to detect the presence of CPV in the stool samples at CADRAD, IVRI, Izatnagar. It has been widely applied to provide rapid, sensitive and accurate diagnosis of the disease. The PCR has been found to detect fewer particles of CPV-2 than other tests like HA and ELISA. The PCR can now be used to differentiate the different mutants (CPV-2, 2a and 2b) of CPV-2 using the primers specific for particular mutants. Either the nested PCR using internal primers or the RE analysis of PCR product of conventional PCR can also be used to further confirm the result of the PCR. The confirmatory diagnosis of the mutants of the CPV responsible for the disease can be ascertained by sequencing the genes coding the structural proteins. The confirmatory diagnosis of the mutants of the CPV-2 responsible for the disease can be ascertained by sequencing the gene coding the structural proteins.

Therapy : The restoration of the electrolyte and fluid balance is the most important goal of therapy. The affected dog should be put under broad spectrum antibiotic umbrella (ampicillin, chloramphenicol, erythromycin, gentamycin etc.). Norfloxacin and nalidixic acid have been proved to be effective against canine haemorrhagic gastroenteritis. The symptomatic treatment with steroid, broad spectrum antibiotic, fluid and electrolyte may save the life of the animal. During the early phase of the disease, the application of hyperimmune serum may help to reduce the virus load and render the infection less dramatic. Such treatment has been shown to reduce the mortality and shorten the length of the disease however hyperimmune serum is difficult to obtain. In case of vomition, Reglan @ 0.5 mg /kg body weight (Metaclopromide) may be given at 8 hours interval. To correct the gastric problem cimetidine, ranitidine, famotidine and to check diarrhea, loparamide or bismuth subnitrate or other astringent preparations may be given. A dog with persistent vomition should not be given any food until diarrhea and vomition subsides.

Immunoprophylactic agents : Effective vaccines are available for the prevention of CPV -2 infection. Both modified live and inactivated parvovirus vaccines have been used to fully susceptible sero-negative pups. Attenuated strains of CPV have been derived by repeated passage of the virus in cell culture. The vaccine virus is shed at much lower titres in the faeces suggesting that the absence of enteritis results from decreased viral replication in the intestine. Experimentally live virus vaccines have been shown to protect dogs for at least 3 years or longer. Inactivated vaccine however, provide only a limited duration of immunity to infection and dogs are protected against disease for several months. For parvoviral prophylaxis, modified live virus (MLV) vaccines have proved to be much more effective than inactivated vaccines. MLV vaccines have been shown to be safer and neither vaccine induced diseases, reversion of virulence or the involvement of vaccine viruses in the generation of new viruses have been confirmed.

There is a strong correlation between HI or serum neutralizing antibody titers and resistance to infection with CPV. The HI test has been useful to measure antibodies which correlated with immunity. The HI titre > 1:40 or 1:80 is considered protective. The highest rate of infection is reported in pups older than 6 weeks of age. As with other infectious diseases of dogs, puppies from immune bitches are protected for the first week of life by maternal antibodies which are acquired via the colostrum. Successful immunization with most vaccines can be accomplished with a high degree of confidence only in seronegative pups, or in pups with very low antibody titers. Maternal antibodies are acquired during the initial 2-3 days of life and then decline, with an average half life of about 9-10 days. Passively acquired antibody titers below 40 are not considered protective against infection but they commonly interfere with immunization. There is a critical period where maternal antibodies are no longer present in sufficient quantity to confer protection, but 90% of the pups from vaccinated populations respond to vaccines at 12 weeks of age.

Vaccination of dogs is generally performed using multivalent vaccines, which contain CDV, CPV, leptospira bacterin and inactivated rabies virus. Monovalent CPV-2 vaccines are also available, some of them containing very high titer (10^7 $TCID_{50}$) and widely recommended for initial vaccination of pups. About 60% of all puppies seroconverted after a single vaccination either at 6 weeks of age with a CPV monovalent vaccine or at 8 weeks of age with a multivalent vaccine. At 12 weeks of age another shot is given when all pups had received 2-3 inoculation at this age but nearly 10% pups still had not sero-converted. The principal reason for the non-responders was the persistence of interfering levels of maternal antibodies. None of the vaccines tested were capable of breaking through a maternal antibody titer of 1:160 or higher, regardless whether the vaccines were high titered or not.

The following general vaccination schedule is recommended.

1. Vaccination at 6 weeks of age with a CPV-2 monovalent vaccine.
2. Vaccination at 8 weeks of age with a multivalent vaccine CPV, CDV, canine adenovirus (CAV), leptospira and rabies antigen.
3. Vaccination at 15 of 16 weeks of age with a multivalent vaccine CPV, CDV, CAV, leptospira and rabies antigen.

If it is necessary to develop an individual vaccination schedule, determination of the antibody titer of one or two pups in the litter could be determined at 5 or 6 weeks of age, then vaccination of the litter may be calculated on the basis of titer, using an estimated antibody half life of 9.5 days. Vaccination is likely to be successful when the maternal antibody titer has declined to less than 1:10. Titer below 1:40 are variably protective, but they may interfere with vaccination.

An attenuated live FPLV vaccine for CPV-2b infection has shown that vaccinated specific pathogen free (SPF) cats are protected from challenge with CPV-2b at 2 weeks after vaccination. However, antibody titers induced by a FPLV vaccine are significantly lower against CPVs than FPLV. It is better to use homologous inactivated vaccines that use CPV-2a or CPV-2b for cats. CPV-2a/CPV-2b based vaccines are expected to protect cats more efficiently from CPV-2 infection than conventional FPLV vaccines. Again, like FPLV vaccine for CPV-2 infection, CPV2a/2b based vaccines may be less efficient for FPLV infection which would be a major concern. Interestingly, CPV-2c infected cats showed similar neutralization antibody titers against FPLV, CPV-2a, CPV- 2b as well as CPV2c . An inactivated CPV-2c based vaccine for cats could be a promising vaccine candidate against both CPV and FPLV infection.

Recombinant vaccine : Recombinant vaccine containing the baculovirus expressed VP2 protein was found to be structurally and immunologically indistinguishable from authentic VP2. The recombinant VP2 also shows the capability to self assemble, forming virus like particles similar in size and appearance to CPV virions. The VP2 protein at the rate of 10 μg was able to elicit good protective response as measured by ELISA and shown to be better than commercially available inactivated CPV vaccine in terms of immune response. The expressed VP2 was administered along with the Quil A (50 μg/ animal), alumina or both adjuvants on 0 day and 28 days to improve the immunogenicity of the vaccine at different doses (10 μg, 25 μg, 50 μg and 100 μg). All the vaccinated dogs maintained the protective antibody response up to 6 days observation period and withstood challenge virus infection 42 days after the booster doses.

DNA vaccines : Both the prokaryotic and eukaryotic vectors harbouring the genes coding for the structural proteins of the canine parvovirus has shown encouraging results. The dogs immunized with the DNA vaccines withstood the challenge with virulent canine parvovirus. However, the DNA vaccines is still in the experimental stage and not yet licensed to be used in the field condition.

Conclusion : Canine parvovirus infections in dogs has been regarded as one of the most important diseases of dogs. Since it was first reported in 1977, the disease has been reported from many countries of the world including India. Although potent and efficacious live attenuated and inactivated vaccines are available in India, large number of cases are diagnosed by HA, HI, ELISA or PCR mostly from the unvaccinated dogs. As the CPV-2 is very resistant to environmental conditions, they remain viable for long period of time in nature. The stray dogs are not vaccinated against the disease and they remain carrier of the virus and source of infection to other susceptible dogs. Extensive studies must be undertaken to know the molecular epidemiology of the canine parvovirus infections in different species and the variants of the CPV involved in the outbreak of the disease. The necessary preventive measures must be undertaken to immunize the susceptible dogs including the stray dogs with potent and efficacious vaccines against the disease to check the spread of the disease.

References

Afshar, A. (1981). Canine parvovirus infections – a review. *Vet Bull.* 51 : 605-612.

Appel, M.J.G., Scott, F.W. and Carmichael, L.E. (1979). Isolation and immunization studies of a canine parvo-like virus from dogs with hemorrhagic enteritis. *Vet. Rec.* 105: 156-159.

Battilani, M., Scagliarini, A., Tisato, E., Turilli, C., Jacoboni, I., Casadio, R. and Prosperi, S. (2001). Analysis of canine parvovirus sequences from wolves and dogs isolated in Italy. *J. Gen. Virol.* 82 : 1555-1560.

Black, J.W., Holscher, M.A., Powell, H.S. and Byerly, C.S. (1979). Parvoviral enteritis and panleucopenia in dogs. *Vet. Med. Small Anim. Clin.* 74: 47-50.

Burtonboy, G.F., Coignoul, N.D. and Pastoret, P.P. (1979). Canine haemorrhagic enteritis: detection of viral particles by electron microscopy. *Arch. Virol.* 61:1-11.

Carmichael, L. (2005). An annotated historical account of canine parvovirus. *J Vet Med. B Infect. Dis. Vet. Pub. Hlth.* 52 (7-8): 303–11.

Carmichael, L.E., Joubert, J.C. and Pollock, R.V. (1993). A modified live canine parvovirus vaccine. II Immune response. *Cornell Vet.* 73: 13-29.

Carpenter, J.L., Roberts, R.M., Harpster, N.K. and King, N.W. (1980). Intestinal and cardiopulmonary forms of parvovirus infection in a litter of pups. *J. Am. Vet. Med. Assoc.* 176: 1269-1273

Cavalli, A., Martella, V., Costantina, D., Michele, C., Bellacicco, A.L., Pasquale, D.P. and Buonavoglia, C. (2004). Evaluation of the antigenic relationships among canine parvovirus type 2 variants. *Clin. Vaccine Immunol.* 15 (3): 534-9.

Fletcher, K.C., Bugster, A.K., Schmidt, R.E. and Hubbard, G.B. (1979). Parvovirus infection in maned wolves. *J. Am. Vet. Med. Assoc.* 175: 897-900.

Glia, G.B., Decaro, G.E.N. and Carmichael, L.E. (2001) Evidence for evolution of canine parvovirus type-2 in Italy. *J. Gen. Virol.* 82:1555-1560.

Greenwood, N.M., Chalmers, W.S.K., Baxendale, W. and Thompson, H. (1995). Comparison of isolates of canine parvovirus by restriction enzyme analysis, and vaccine efficacy against field strains. *Vet Rec.* 136:63–67.

Gupta, P.K., Rai, A., Rai, N., Raut, A.A. and Chauhan, S. (2005). Cloning of canine parvovirus VP2 gene and its use as DNA vaccine in dogs. *Current Science.* 88: 778-782.

Hirasawa, T., Kaneshige, T. and Mikazuki, K. (1994). Sensitive detection of canine parvovirus DNA by the nested PCR. *Vet. Microbiol.* 41: 135-145.

Houston, D.M., Ribble, C.S. and Head, L.L. (1996). Risk factors associated with parvovirus enteritis in dogs. *J. Am. Vet. Med. Assoc.* 208: 542-548.

Hueffer, K., Govindasamy, L.,. Agbandje-McKenna, M. and Parrish, C.R. (2003). Combinations of two capsid regions controlling canine host range determine canine transferrin receptor binding by canine and feline parvoviruses. *J. Virol.* 77:10099–10105.

Ikeda, Y., Mochizuki, M., Naito, R., Nakamura, K., Miyazawa, T., Mikami, T. and Takahashi, E. (2000). Predominance of canine parvovirus (CPV) in unvaccinated cat populations and emergence of new antigenic types of CPVs in cats. *J. Virol.* 278 : 13-19.

Khadilkar, M.V., Batra, P. and Singhvi, N.M. (1994). A suspected outbreak of myocardial form of canine parvovirus in army dogs. *J. Rem. Vet. Corps.* 33: 73-79.

Kramer, J.M., Meunter, P.C. and Pollock, R.V.H. (1980). Canine parvovirus: update. *Vet. Med. Small Anim. Clin.* 175: 1541-1555.

Lopez de Turiso, J.A., Cortes, E., Ranz, A., Garcia, J., Sanz, A., Vela, C. and. Casal, J.I. (1991). Fine mapping of canine parvovirus B cell epitopes. *J. Gen. Virol.* 72: 2445–2456.

Lopez de Turiso, J.A., Cortes, E., Martinez, C., Vela, C. and Casal, J.I. (1992). Recombinant vaccine for canine parvovirus in dogs. *J. Virol.* 66: 2748-2753.

Mochizuki, M., Horiuchi, M., Hiragi, H., San Gabriel, M.C., Yasuda, N. and Uno, T. (1996). Isolation of canine parvovirus from a cat manifesting clinical signs of feline panleucopenia. *J. Clin. Microbiol.* 34: 2101-2105.

Murphy, F.A., Fauquet, C.M. and Bishop, D.H.L. (1995). Parvoviridae. In: Virus taxonomy. Sixth report of the International Committee on Taxonomy of Viruses, pp. 169–178. Springer-Verlag Wien, New York, NY.

Murphy, F.A., Gibbs, E.P.J., Horzinek. M.C. and Studdert, M.J. (1999). Parvoviridae. In: Veterinary virology, 3rd ed., pp. 343–356. San Diego, CA.,

Nandi, S., Pandey, A.B., Sharma, K., Audarya, S.D. and Chauhan, R.S. (2007). Development and standardization of PCR for the detection of Canine Parvoviral DNA in the stool samples of canines. Fourth Convention of Society for Immunology and Immunopathology and National Symposium on Immunobiotechnology and Workshop on "Molecular and Immunological Methods in the diagnosis of Tuberculosis" held at Tuberculosis Research Centre and Madras Veterinary College, Chennai, from Feb 25-27, 2007.

Nandi, S. and Sinha, D. K. (2002). Evolution and emergence of canine parvovirus variants – a real problem. *The Veterinarian.* 26: 12-14.

Nandi, S., Anbazhagan, R. and Pandey, A.B. (2005). PCR based diagnosis of different variants of canine parvovirus in vaccines and field samples. International Congress of Canine Practice and Symposium on Emerging Changes in Canine Practice organized by organized by Indian Society for Advancement of Canine Practice (ISACP) held at Hotel Hyatt Regency, New Delhi from February 9-11, 2005.

Nandi, S., Audarya, S.D., Suresh, I . and Chauhan, R.S. (2006). Canine Parvovirus Infection in Dogs – a Challenge to Veterinary Community. Lead paper presented in Short Term Training Course on *Laboratory Diagnosis of Animal Diseases and Zoonoses.* 172-182.

Nandi, S., Pandey, A.B., Sharma, K. and Chauhan, R.S. (2008). Polymerase chain reaction for the detection of canine parvoviral DNA in vaccines. *Indian J. Virol.* 19 (1) : 9-11.

Nelson, D.T., Eustis, S.L., McAdaragh, J.P and Stotz, I. (1979). Lesions of spontaneous canine viral enteritis. *Vet. Path,* 16: 680-686.

Parrish, C.R., Aquadro, C.F., Strassheim, M.L., Evermann, J.F., Sgro, J.Y. and Mohammed, H.O. (1991). Rapid antigenic type replacement and DNA sequence evolution of canine parvovirus. *J. Virol.* 65: 6544-6552

Parrish, C.R. and Kawaoka, Y. (2005). The origins of new pandemic viruses: the acquisition of new host ranges by canine parvovirus and influenza A viruses. *Annu. Rev. Microbiol.* 59: 553–586.

Pereira, C.A., Monezi, T.A., Mehnert, D.U., D'Angelo, M. and Durigon, E.L. (2000). Molecular characterization of canine parvovirus in Brazil by PCR. *Vet. Microbiol.* 75: 127-133.

Pratelli, A., Cavalli, A., Normanno, G., De Palma, G.M., Buonavoglia, C. and Martella, V. (2000). Immunization of pups with maternally derived antibodies to canine parvovirus (CPV) using a modified-live variant (CPV-2b). *J. Vet. Med.* 47: 273–276.

Robinson, W.F., Huxtable, C.R. and Pass, D.A. (1980). Canine parvoviral myocarditis: a morphological description of the natural disease. *Vet. Path.* 17: 282-293.

Sagazio, P., Tempesta, M., Buonavoglia, D., Cirone, F. and Buonavoglia, C. (1998). Antigenic characterization of canine parvovirus strains isolated in Italy. *J. Virol. Meth.* 73 : 197-200.

Scott, F.W. (1980). Vircucidal disinfectants and feline viruses. *Am. J. Vet. Res.* 41: 410-414.

Siegl, G. (1976). The parvoviruses. *Virol. Monogr.* 15: 1-109

Spibey, N., Greenwood, N.M., Sutton, D., Chalmers, W.S. and Tarpey, I.(2008). Canine parvovirus type 2 vaccine protects against virulent challenge with type 2c virus. *Vet. Microbiol.* 128 (1-2): 48-55

Stann, S.E., DiGiacomo, R.F., Giddens, W.E. and Evermann, J.F. (1984). Clinical and pathological features of parvoviral diarrhoea in dogs. *J. Am. Vet. Med. Assoc.* 185: 651.

Tratschin, J.D., McMaster, G.K., Kronauer, G. and Siegl, G. (1982). Canine parvovirus relationship to wild-type and vaccine strains of feline panleucopenia virus and mink enteritis virus. *J. Gen. Virol.* 61: 33-41.

Truyen, U., Platzer, G. and Parrish, C.R. (1996). Antigenic type distribution among canine parvoviruses in dogs and cats in Germany. *Vet. Rec.* 138: 365-366.

Waner, T., Naveh, A., Wudovsky, I. and Carmichael, L.E. (1996). Assessment of maternal antibody decay and response to canine parvovirus vaccination using a clinic-based enzyme linked immunosorbent assay. *J. Vet. Diagn. Invest.* 8: 427–432.

Waner, T., Mazar, S., Nachmias, E., Keren-Kornblatt, E. and Harrus, S. (2003). Evaluation of a dot ELISA kit for measuring immunoglobulin M antibodies to canine parvovirus and distemper virus. *Vet. Rec.* 152:588– 591.

Woods, C.B., Pollock, R.V.H. and Carmichael, L.E. (1980).Canine parvoviral enteritis. *J. Am. Anim. Hosp. Assoc.* 16: 171-179.

B. Bacterial Diseases

11

Black Quarter

Synonyms : Black leg, quarter ill

This is an acute infectious but non contagious disease of cattle, goat, sheep, swine and deer caused by *Cl. chauvoei* characterized by development of focal gangrenous and emphysematous myositis. This gives rise to crepitation and serosanguinous swelling in heavy muscles especially in gluteal muscles and associated with severe toxaemia and high mortality.

Etiology : B.Q is caused by *Cl. chauvoei*, a Gm positive rod shaped motile, spore forming toxin producing anaerobes. They are 0.6 μ in diameter and 3 to 8 μ in length. The spores are placed terminally or subterminally and very much resistant to altered environmental stress. The spores are very much unaffected to hot desiccation and disinfectants. Spores can persist in the soil for number of years and withstand 120ºC for 10 min. The organisms can be destroyed by 3% formalin in 15 min and by 2% bichloride of Hg in 10 min. False BQ may be caused by *Cl. septicum* and *Cl. novyi*. *Cl. chauvoei* exists as one biotype and it is serologically homogenous whereas *Cl. septicum* has got 4 major antigenic groups.

Distribution : The disease is widespread in most of the tropical countries of the world. In India the disease is sporadic in nature and reported from all the states of the countries during rainy season.

Susceptible hosts : Cattle are the most susceptible host but may occur in sheep, buffalo, goat, deer and rarely in pigs. Cattle of 4 to 24 months of age group and having good body condition are more susceptible.

Mode of transmission : The disease spreads from soils contaminated with infected carcasses. Animals are infected through ingestion of infected feeds possibly through contamination of wounds. The normal healthy animals may harbour bacteria in the spleen, liver and alimentary tract and excrete the organisms through faeces. In sheep, the bacteria is introduced through shearing, docking, lambing, castration and in rare instances following vaccination against enterotoxaemia. Guinea pigs can be infected experimentally.

Pathogenesis : It is chiefly a pastoral disease and mostly occurs in wet weather spells during spring and autumn while grazing on low lying pastures. Ingested organisms are carried from the intestine via circulation to the skeletal muscles. Welformed muscles of gluteal region, loin, shoulder are affected. There is necrosis of the muscles fibers due to fermentation. The muscles of the tongue, jaw, heart may be affected at a later stage. Highly virulent organisms produce potent exotoxin causing high temperature, rapid respiration, degenerative changes, local necrotizing myositis and a fatal systemic toxaemia. Severe toxemia may lead to death.

Clinical signs : Cattle : The incubation period is 2-5 days and the course of the disease is 24 to 60 h. The rise of temperature up to 106-108°F with lameness are the early symptoms. The characteristic swelling develops in one of the thick layers of muscles such as thigh, buttocks, shoulder, necks and lumber region. Swellings are hot and painful in the early stage and become cold and painless later. The muscle tissues are swollen, dark in color and turn dry. On pressure swellings emit cracking or crepitation sound due to emphysema. When the swelling is incised a reddish exudate escapes from the wound giving off a rancid colour. Regional lymph nodes are swollen. The appetite is lost and rumination is suppressed with recumbency, dyspnoea and thready pulse. Temperature falls just before the death of the animal.

Sheep : There is haemorrhagic oedema in the S/C tissues following a wound. Animals show loss of appetite, fever, prostration and death. Lameness may be present but not a constant feature.

Horse : The oedema of the pectoral muscles, stiffness of gait and ataxia have been observed.

Lesions : Lesions are observed mainly in muscles of shoulder, thigh and neck but tongue, diaphragm and myocardium may be affected. Large crepitating swellings are the most characteristic necropsy findings. Affected muscles are infiltrated with yellowish exudate with gas bubbles. A rancid odour emanates from the muscle and there is accumulation of fluid in the pericardium. The conjunctival mucous membrane become congested. The liver, kidney, lungs and spleen show yellowish foci and haemorrhage. Blood stained discharge may ooze from the natural orifice.

Microscopically affected muscles show coagulative necrosis, infiltration of leukocytes and haemolysis of erythrocytes. Gm + rods are noted throughout the lesions.

Diagnosis : The tentative diagnosis is made from the history, clinical signs and post mortem lesions.

Microscopical examination of smear : The examination of smear from the affected tissues or fluids of the swellings reveal Gm+ rods with subterminal spores. Sometimes *Cl. chauvoei* and *Cl. septicum* may occur as mixed infection. Therefore specific isolation and identification of *Cl. chauvoei* should be made.

Cultural isolation : Anaerobic media provides growth within 24 h and materials to be used are heart blood, peritoneal fluids and affected muscles.

Biological test : Muscle pieces from the lesions are in sterile saline and filtrate containing spores are heated to 60oC for 30 min. 1 ml is injected into the gluteal muscles of guinea pigs. In positive cases where the materials contain spores of *Cl. chauvoei,* the animals die within 48 h. The impression smear of infected tissues reveal Gram positive rods having subterminal spores.

Differential diagnosis : B.Q. must be differentiated from anthrax, malignant oedema and bacillary haemoglobinuria. Anthrax and bacillary haemoglobinuria may be enzootic in some places and may occur at any season of the year with symptoms of bloat and bloody discharges. But S/C crepitation and local swellings are absent. B.Q. must not be confused with sweet clover poisoning, a nonfebrile, non-transmissible disease of cattle occurs in the gluteal, costal or shoulder regions with large amount of blood. They pit on pressure and crepitation is absent.

Treatment : In advanced stage of the disease, treatment is of no use. Penicillin, aureomycin and oxytetracycline may be injected into the affected muscles. Penicillin @ 10,000 I.U. /Kg B.Wt may be used. Crystalline Penicillin may be used through I/V route followed by procaine Penicillin through I/M route for 7-9 days. New antibiotic cephaloridine may be tried.

Control : Since the disease is associated with infection from the soil, the young animals should be kept out of such area. The skin of the dead body should not be taken out and it should be burnt or buried. The animals should not be allowed to graze in endemic pasture. All the animals of the endemic zones should be vaccinated with suitable vaccine.

Immunization : The most reliable method of preventing losses from BQ is by means of vaccinating all cattle and sheep between the age of 6 to 24 months of age. In enzootic areas, vaccination is carried out when the incidence of the disease is very high usually summer and before the onset of monsoon. Vaccination of calves at 3 weeks of age when the risk is very high followed by revaccination at 6 months of age. Following vaccines are used.

(i) Cl. chauvoei, Cl. septicum and *P. multocida vaccine* : This vaccine is available for protecting the animals against B.Q and HS simultaneously.

(ii) BQ vaccine (polyvalent) : This vaccine is given S/C in cattle and other ruminant animals for prophylaxis against malignant oedema. Dose is 5 ml in cattle and buffalo, 2-3 ml in sheep and goat. Booster dose is given 10 days later, immunity develops within a fortnight and lasts for 1 year.

(iii) Combined HS and BQ vaccine : It is a combined vaccine containing *P. multocida* type I and *Cl. chauvoei* respectively. It protects against both the disease. Dose is 5 ml S/C in case of cattle and buffaloes.

Young animals are vaccinated at 6 months of age and immunity lasts for one year.

Passive immunization : Immune serum @ 40-60-100 ml (add 20 ml every hour) until temperatures subsides.

Further reading

Awad, F.I., Farrag, I. and Hussein, A.Z. (1986). The immunizing power of three blackleg vaccines. *Assiut Vet Med J.* 17: 201-211.

Awad, F.I., Gadalla, M.S. and Farrag, I. (1973). Studies on the aetiology of black quarter in Egyptian cattle. *Egyptian J Vet Sci.* 10: 45-51.

Chakraborti, A. (2000). Black quarter. *A Textbook of Preventive Veterinary Medicine*, pp 375-381. Kalyani Publishers, New Delhi.

Merchant, I.A. and Packer, R.A. (1983). The genus *Clostridium. Veterinary Bacteriology and Virology*, 7th edn, pp 389-402. CBS Publisher & Distributor, New Delhi.

Noble, J. (2007). Cattle diseases: Blackleg. Available at: *http:// www2. dpi.qld. gov. au/ beef/ 3450.html.* Accessed 22 August 2007.

Radostits, O.M., Gay, C. C., Hinchcliff, K.W. and Constable, P.D. (2007). Veterinary Medicine : A Textbook of the diseases of Cattle, Horses, Sheep, Pigs and Goats, 10th edn., Philadelphia, Elsevier Saunders. 2007.

Robson S. 2007. Blackleg in cattle. Available at: *http:// www.thedairysite.com/ articles /843/blackleg-in-cattle*. Accessed 22 August 2007.

Samad, M .A. (2001). Bacterial disease. *Animal Husbandry and Medicine*, 2nd edn, pp 599-601. LEP Publication, Dhaka.

Udall, D.H. (1972). Acute bacterial disease. *The Practice of Veterinary Medicine*, 6th edn, pp 430-435. Oxford & IBH Publishing Co Pvt Ltd, Andra Pradesh.

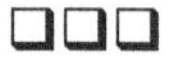

12

Bovine Tuberculosis

Synonymous : Pearl's disease, scrofula

It is a chronic insidious contagious disease of man and animals caused by tubercle bacilli characterized by development of tubercles in lung tissue, lymph nodes or other organs resulting in caseation and calcification. The tubercles are frequently located in lungs and lymph nodes. But they may be formed in the liver, spleen, intestine, peritoneum, meninges and long bones. It is a zoonotic disease. Bovine tuberculosis, caused by *Mycobacterium bovis* (*M. bovis*) is considered as the serious epizootics of animals and humans. Bovine species are natural hosts to the disease, but a wide spectrum of domestic and wild animals, as well as man, can be infected. Animals reported as having been infected with *M. bovis* include North American bison (*Bison bison*), buffaloes (*Syncerus caffer*), elk (*Cervus elaphus*), domestic and wild pigs (*Sus scrofa*), goats (*Capra hircus*), camels (*Camelus bactrianus*), dogs (*Canis familiaris*), cats (*Felis catus*), sheep (*Ovis aries*), possums (*Trichosurus vulpecula*), badgers (*Meles meles*), mink (*Lutreola vison*), ferrets (*Putorius furo*) and non-human primates. All species are not equally susceptible, and are often grouped into spill-over (end) hosts and maintenance hosts. Cattle and other bovine species are considered the primary and most well-known reservoirs or maintenance hosts. In countries where maintenance hosts are present endemically in the wild, infection from these populations to domestic cattle or other farm animals is difficult to avoid. In Africa, bovine TB primarily affects cattle ; however, infection in other farm and domestic animals, such as sheep, goats, pigs, dogs and cats, is not uncommon. Wild ruminants and carnivores are also affected and are the natural reservoirs of the infectious agent in the wild. Man is also susceptible to the disease, the highest risk groups being individuals with concomitant HIV/AIDS infection. In Africa, human TB is widely known to be caused by *M. tuberculosis*; however, an unknown proportion of cases are due to *M. bovis.* This infection in humans is underreported as a result of the diagnostic limitations of many laboratories in distinguishing *M. bovis* from *M. tuberculosis.* TB is a neglected public health problem and accounts for about 25% of all avoidable adult deaths in developing countries. It is of socio-economic significance, as it can affect international trade in animals and animal products. Many factors account for the failure of developing countries to control and eradicate bovine TB, many of them politico-economic. Added to the high costs of a sustainable testing programme are problems of social unrest due to political instability and ethnic wars, resulting in the displacement of large numbers of human and animal populations; lack of veterinary expertise and communication networks; insufficient collaboration with bordering countries and hence a lack of quarantine; and smuggling of live animals across state boundaries. Scarce human and financial resources are often absorbed by action against the high incidence of other acute and fatal diseases, such as contagious bovine pleuropneumonia, foot and mouth disease, African and classical swine fever and parasitic diseases. The primary sources of infection for humans are consumption of unpasteurised milk and close association between humans and animals. Rural inhabitants and some urban dwellers in Africa still consume unpasteurised and soured milk potentially infected with *M. bovis*. Milk-borne infection is the main cause of non-pulmonary TB in areas where bovine TB is common and uncontrolled.

Etiology : Bovine TB is caused by *M. bovis*. Although cattle are considered to be the primary hosts of *M. bovis*, the disease has an exceptionally wide mammalian host range, which includes humans. *M. bovis* is a member of a closely related group of mycobacteria referred to as Mycobacterium Tuberculosis Complex (MTC), which comprises *M. tuberculosis*, *M. africanum*, *M. bovis*, *M. microti* and *M. bovis*. Isolates with characteristics intermediate between *M. tuberculosis* and *M. bovis* have also been reported. MTC bacteria are usually regarded as subspecies and are characteristically 99.9% similar at the nucleotide level, with identical 16S rRNA sequences. However, there are distinct phenotypic differences between the subspecies, and not host range and pathogenicity. *M. bovis* closely resembles *M. tuberculosis*, and precise identification of and distinction between the two can be established by biochemical and molecular biology techniques. In the public health centres of most developing countries, Löwenstein-Jensen (LJ) medium, a medium on which *M. bovis* may grow poorly or not at all, is commonly used for the isolation of *M. tuberculosis*. Inoculated media are often incubated insufficiently for *M. bovis* cultures to appear. This may help to explain the low number of bovine type human TB cases reported in developing countries. *M. bovis* is a robust pathogen and may survive in the environment, in buildings, on transport vehicles, on pasture and in slurry. The organism has been reported to survive in cow faeces for more than 5 months in winter, 4 months in autumn, 2 months in summer, and in soil for up to 2 years. Manure fertilisation of arable land is common practice in developing countries; survival of *M. bovis* in soil and slurry therefore implies pasture and vegetable contamination, representing a potential source of infection to animals and humans, respectively.

Distribution : It is an ancient disease and worldwide in distribution. The disease is highly prevalent in the tropical and subtropical countries. The disease has been eradicated from Canada, Denmark, Finland, Germany, Great Britain, Switzerland, USA and USSR by systemic application of tuberculin test and removal of all animals showing positive reactions. In India, it is endemic and has been recorded from all the states.

Epidemiology : All species including humans and age groups are susceptible to *M. bovis* with cattle, goats and pigs most susceptible and sheep and horses showing high natural resistance. Cattle are most susceptible and bovine strains is most pathogenic over the three strains. Incidence is more in pure bred and cross bred cattle. Zebu cattle are relatively resistant to bovine tuberculosis. Tuberculosis occurs in most of the country of the world and is of major importance in dairy cattle. Apart from actual death, animals lose 10-25% of their productive efficiency. In England and Ireland infected badgers (*Meles meles*) are significant in the epidemiology of the disease and infection of cattle is believed to be from badger's urine contamination of pastures, farm building and cattle troughs. In New Zealand cattle can get infection from brush tail possum (*Trichosurus vulpecula*) having lesions in peripheral lymph nodes with discharging sinuses during contact in bush and pasture. Mule deer (*Odocoileus hemionus*), white tailed deer (*O. virginianus*), elk (*Cervus elaphus canadensis*) and bison (*Bison bison*) in N. America and red deer in Great Britain and Ireland can act as maintenance host and some regions spread infection to cattle. Buffaloes (*Syncerys caffer*) in S. Africa and water buffaloes (*Bubalis bubalis*) in Australia can also act as maintenance host in those countries.

Pathogenesis : The capacity of tuberculous organisms to elicit a disease depends on complex lipids present in their cell wall (trehalose -6-6' dimycolate) or strongly acidic lipids. These toxic lipids released by virulent tubercle baclli initiates disruption of phagosome, interfere with phagolysosome formation, alter the release of hydrolytic enzymes form the lysomes and inactivate the lysosomal enzymes released into the cytoplasmic vacuoles.

There are numerous ways in which cattle can become infected with *M. bovis*; these can be affected by animal age and behaviour, environment and climate, and prevailing farming practices. Under natural conditions, the main route of *M. bovis* infection in cattle is by inhalation. This mode of transmission is dominant in industrialised countries, where intensive farming is practised. In field case studies of bovine TB in these countries, lesion distribution and pathology show predominant involvement of the upper and lower respiratory tract and associated lymph nodes. Confirmed tuberculin reactors frequently appear to have an absence of lung lesions; however, lesions when present within the lung parenchyma are usually too small (1cm) to be easily detected during meat inspection. A generally accepted concept is that infection with *M. bovis* can become established in cattle by inhalation of tubercle bacilli, possibly a single bacillus, in an aerosol droplet that lodges within the respiratory tract, probably the alveolar surface of the lung. Bacilli are phagocytosed by macrophages, and subsequently interact with cells involved in innate and acquired immune responses in tissue or draining lymph nodes. This often results in nonvascular nodular granulomas known as 'tubercles'. Characteristic tuberculous lesions occur most frequently in lungs and retropharyngeal, bronchial and mediastinal lymph nodes. Lesions can also be found in the mesenteric lymph nodes, liver, spleen, serous membranes, pleura and other organs. The role of activated mononuclear macrophages is considered most important in protecting the host against *M. bovis.* Macrophages are involved in processing mycobacterial antigens and presenting them to T-lymphocytes, which are considered a key recognition unit in the immune response to mycobacteria. The characteristic lesion caused by *M. bovis* in cattle is described as having a centre of caseous necrosis, usually with some calcification, with a boundary of epithelioid cells, some of which form multinucleated giant cells and few to numerous lymphocytes and neutrophils. Primary lesions in cattle, unlike man, are rarely contained by the immune response, and dissemination from a lesion may occur by natural ducts such as bronchi, by lymphatic spread or by haematogenous spread when massive miliary TB occurs. It is worth noting that despite the many studies on bovine TB over the years, it was recently concluded that a better understanding of the dynamics of the events following *M. bovis* exposure of cattle and subsequent infection would be of significant benefit to diagnosis and disease control.

Transmission : Young animals are less susceptible whereas younger human beings are more susceptible to tuberculosis. Malnourished animals readily contract the infection rather than well nourished group. Vitamin C and A deficiency predispose the infection. Overcrowding house and premises and common drinking and feeding troughs are the important sources of disease transmission. Poor sanitation and poor ventilation are the contributory factors for the entry and establishment of the disease. Infected animals excrete the organisms in the exhaled air, in sputum, faeces, milk, urine, vaginal and uterine and wound discharges. Susceptible animals contract the infection directly through contact with tuberculous animals or their discharges. Faeces of cattle have been found to remain infective for 6-8 weeks in slurry. Disease may be transmitted through contaminated instruments or utensils. Cattle may be infected while they come in contact with tuberculous people or animals. Cattle may acquire the infection from infected cattle handler and vice versa. Calves get infected via infected milk. Disease is mostly prevalent in farmed dairy cattle rather than free range cattle due to overcrowding. Carnivorous animals often pick up the infection from inhalation of infected meat/milk. Pigs pick up the infection through milk or cow dung. The cows may be infected through infected bulls or A.I. with infected semen.

Zebu cattle (*Bos indicus*) are more resistant to tuberculous than European cattle and effect on this cattle are much severe. Goats are quite susceptible and sheep are relatively resistant. In horses the disease occurs rarely.

Inhalation of *M. bovis* is the most probable and principal route to bovine infection and is facilitated by close, prolonged contact between infected and healthy animals. Ingestion of *M. bovis* directly from infected animals or from contaminated pasture, water or utensils may also be very common in some regions. While congenital infections and vertical transmission have been recorded, these routes, like genital transmission, which occurs when reproductive organs are infected, are now rarely seen in regions that have intensive eradication programmes.

Animal-to-animal transmission : Infectious animals may shed *M. bovis* in a number of ways: in faeces, milk, discharging lesions, saliva and urine. Intensive livestock farming promotes close contact between animals, favouring the spread of *M. bovis.* Close contact between animals occurs for example at water points such as ponds, wells and streams. Vaccination and artificial insemination centres, dipping tanks, auction stations, market places and transportation are the commonest animal gathering places, and again are sites where transmission of infection could easily occur. Possibly the most dangerous spots for nose-to-nose or mouth-to-mouth contact between animals are salt supplementing points. Therefore, while extensive farming is safer than zero level grazing systems to prevent disease transmission, some of the above situations simulate the dangers of intensive farming in relation to disease transmission.

Animal-to-human transmission : Human TB due to *M. bovis* in developing countries today is analogous to conditions in the 1930s and 1940s in Europe, where more than 50% of cervical lymphadenitis cases in children were caused by *M. bovis* infection. This is exacerbated by the added burden of HIV/acquired immune-deficiency syndrome (AIDS). In industrialised countries, the incidence of TB due to *M. bovis* in humans is almost at zero level as a result of pasteurisation of milk and milk products and eradication of bovine TB in cattle populations. However, in developing countries, bovine TB in animals can be widely distributed in regions where control measures are not applied or are conducted sporadically and pasteurisation is rarely practised. In industrialised countries, the direct correlation between *M. bovis* in cattle and TB due to *M. bovis* in humans has been well documented, whereas little information is available from developing countries. Pulmonary TB due to *M. bovis* is more common in rural dwellers, as a result of inhalation of dust particles or bacteria-containing aerosols shed by infected animals, while urban dwellers acquire the infection via the gastrointestinal route and develop extra-pulmonary TB. In countries with a relatively high prevalence of bovine TB in cattle, abattoir and farm workers are the groups most exposed to infection. Current economic and social globalisation has created greater opportunities for the spread of zoonotic diseases such as TB.

Human-to-animal transmission : The genitourinary tract in humans is a site of non-pulmonary TB due to *M. bovis* ; genitourinary TB may appear to be of little importance to epidemiologists in studying human infection, but this route of infection from man to cattle is well-documented. Farm workers urinating in cowsheds may represent a source of infection for animals. An analogous situation is thought to occur in rural Africa, where patients with genitourinary TB may urinate on pasture: animals craving salt preferentially graze on this grass and may succumb to infection.

Clinical signs : Cattle : The incubation period in natural infection is very long extending from months up to years before any indication of the existence is presented. The insidious nature of the disease, the variability of lesions produced, the variable symptoms produced not only in different species but also in different individual of same species. It is a chronic disease and infected animals lose body weight slowly but continuously in spite of provision of optimum nutrition. Respiratory system is most commonly infected with manifestation of dyspnoea, increased rate of respiration and persistent, painful, dry and hacking cough. The breadth has a foul odour and a mucopurulent material is periodically discharged from the nose and mouth. The respiration is accelerated and frequently accompanied by groaning and grunting. Tuberculous pneumonia and pleurisy may occur. When the disease has extended to the pericardium, there is always marked interference with the action of the heart leading to rope like distension of the jugular vein.

The involvement of the G.I. tract is characterized by abdominal pain, diarrhoea, chronic bloat and emaciation. The faeces is coated with mucous, pus cells and occasionally blood. Constipation followed by diarrhoea and enlargement of mesenteric lymph nodes may be the usual features.

The reproductive disorders include peritonitis, metritis, bursitis and salpingitis. There may be infertility or abortion late in the pregnancy. Lesions similar to those of brucellosis occur on the placenta. There may be a chronic purulent discharge heavily infected with the organism. The testicles if involved are swollen and painful with signs of orchitis and epididymitis.

Tubeculous mastitis is of major public health importance and disease may be spread to calves. Its characteristic feature is marked induration and hypertrophy which usually develops first in the upper part of the udder particularly in the rear quarters. There may be formation of small nodules in the mammary tissue and enlargement of supramammary lymph nodes. On progression of the disease processes, the milk secretion gradually diminishes and ultimately may completely cease. In the early stages the milk is not macroscopically abnormal but very fine floccules appear later and on standing leaving a clear amber fluid.

CNS may be infected and there is impairment or loss of vision, incoordination of gait, hyperesthesia and occasional circling.

Horse : The commonest syndrome in horses is caused by involvement of the cervical vertebrae with painful osteomyelitis, stiffness of the neck and inability to eat off the ground. Less common signs are polyuria, coughing due to pulmonary lesions, lymph node enlargement, nasal discharge and a fluctuating temperature.

Pig : There is enlargement of submaxillary , pharyngeal and cervical lymph node without any clinical abnormality unless they rupture to the exterior. Generalised cases are similar to cattle although tuberculous involvement of the meninges and joints is more common.

Sheep and goat : Bronchopneumonia is the commonest form of the disease manifested by cough and dyspnoea. Some sheep and goats may develop diarrhoea and ulceration of G.I. tract mucosa with fluctuation of temperature. In both the species the disease is slowly progressive but in kids it may be rapidly progressive with early death.

Dog : Dogs may remain as asymptomatic carrier for long period and may be either pulmonary or extrapulmonary type.

Pulmonary type is characterized by characterized by dyspnoea, tachypnoea, chronic cough, pleural and pericardial effusion and pneumothorax. In extrapulmonary form, the kidney, liver and intestine are affected. Faeces with blood and enlargement of liver are evident. Lymph nodes are enlarged.

Cat : T.B. is a rare disease in cats. The clinical manifestation are akin to dogs. They may be infected with bovine or avian strain but resistant to human strain. S/C tuberculous abscess may be formed.

Lesions : Cattle, sheep and goat : The tubercular organisms may affect any tissue or organ. But, lung, liver, pleura, peritoneum, kidney, spleen and regional lymph nodes are commonly affected. In some cases, joints and CNS are affected. Males and female genital organs are also affected occasionally. Uterine, ovarian and testicular lesions are haematogenous in origin but lesions of the penis, vulva and vagina are due to venereal spread.

Tuberculous lesions consist of caseous core surrounded by necrotic tissues and the entire mass is encapsulated with fibrous tissue. The caseous portions may become calcified. The lesions may be large and involve the entire lungs or liver or small or numerous. Such conditions are called milliary T.B. Lesions in bovine T.B. are mostly prevalent in the organs of thoracic cavity rather than abdominal cavity. When the abdominal region is affected the most likely sites are liver, kidney, spleen, intestinal tract and associated lymph nodes. Lesions of kidney, liver and spleen are mostly observed during P.M. examination or meat inspection. Tuberculous lesions may persist in the animals for entire life span and old lesions are usually encapsulated by a much thicker wall of fibrous tissues.

Horse : Large tumour like growths appear in the pharyngeal, mesenteric, cervical and mediastinal lymph nodes. Lungs and bronchial lymph glands are affected and nodules of various sizes are formed in the pulmonary tissues. Lesions in the liver and spleen appear as relatively hard caseous nodules and testis may show ulcerative changes.

Pig : In pig, the pharyngeal lymph nodes are most commonly affected whereas cervical, mediastinal and mesenteric lymph nodes are less commonly affected. In advanced cases affected glands become large tumours like with caseous purulent materials. Lesions may develop in vertebrae, rib, long bones, lung, liver and kidney.

Dog : Both thoracic and abdominal viscera are affected. Small nodules on lungs release milky or straw colour fluid on incision. Miliary to large fibrous nodules are seen in the liver, kidney, intestine and associated lymph glands.

Economics : T.B. occurs in every country of the world and is of major importance in dairy cattle. Apart from actual death, animals lose 10-25% of their productive efficiency.

Zoonotic importance : *M. bovis* can be responsible for 5-10% of human T.B. with higher rates in children. It occurs mainly through consumption of raw milk or milk products. Transmission to humans can be significantly reduced by pasteurization of milk.

Diagnosis : TB can be diagnosed clinically, but usually only in the later stages of the disease. The tuberculin skin test (TST) is universally recognised and is generally used for preliminary diagnosis in bovine TB control programmes. However, in countries with low disease prevalence or disease free status, meat inspection is used for diagnosis and surveillance. Other tests, such as an antibody enzyme-linked immunoassay (ELISA) and the gamma-interferon assay, have been used as supplementary tests in eradication and control. Assays for bovine interferon-gamma have recently been applied to indicate infection. Confirmation of infection, however, often relies on isolation and identification of *M. bovis.*

1. Single intradermal (SID) test : This test is applied by the I/D injection of bovine tuberculin PPD and subsequent detection of swelling as a result of DTH. The tuberculin is prepared from cultures of *M. tuberculosis* or *M. bovis.* Bovine tuberculin is more specific and potent. The reaction is read between 48-72 h for maximum sensitivity and at 96 h for maximum specificity with a diffuse swelling at the injection site. In England and Europe, the injection is made into the cervical fold whereas in US, Canada and Australia and New Zealnad it is the caudal fold of the tail. The cervical fold test is thought to provide greater sensitivity, the caudal fold provides greater specificity. In US 0.1 ml is recommended for herds of unknown status and 0.2 ml for known infected herds when cases with low sensitivity are to be carefully sought. However, the main disadvantage of the SID test is its lack of specificity and number of no visible lesion (NVL) reactors which occur. A maximum permissible rate of 10% is accepted. Further mammalian tuberculinis not sufficiently specific to differentiate between reactions due to infection with *M. bovis* and infection with *M. avium, M. tuberculosis*, *M. paratuberculosis* or *Nocardia farcinicus*. Other disadvantages of the SID test include failure to detect cases of minimum sensitivity such as early and late stages of the disease in old cows and cows recently calved.

1a. Single intradermal (SID) test in pigs : 0.1 ml of mammalian tuberculin is injected into a fold of skin at the base of the ear. The test is read 24-48 h later and a skin thickness of 5 mm or more constitutes a positive reaction. If the animal is infected with *M. avium* and avian tuberculin alone is used the test should be read as 48-72 h and an increase in skin thickness of 4 mm is classed as positive.

1b. Single intradermal (SID) test in horse : 0.1 ml of PPD tuberculin is sufficient to elicit a positive reaction and sometimes anaphylactic reaction. Horses are much more sensitive than cattle to tuberculin. False positive reaction may occur in advanced cases of disease or in old animals due to presence of non-pathogenic organisms.

2. Short thermal test : Intradermal tuberculin (4 ml) is injected S/C into the neck of cattle which have a rectal temperature of not more than 39°C (102°F) at the time of injection and for 2 h later. If the temperature at 4, 6, and 8 h after injection rises above 40°C (104°F), the animal is classed as positive reactor. The temperature peak is usually at 6-8 h and is generally over 41° C (105.8°F). Occasionally death due to anaphylaxis is occur at the peak of reaction.

3. Stormont test : This is a modification of I/D test. 0.1 ml of tuberculin is injected in the neck with a second injection at the same site 7 days later. An increase in the skin thickness of 5 mm or more 24 h after the second injection is a positive result. The increased sensitivity begins at the 5th day, is at its peak at the 7th and ends on the 12th day after the injection. Cattle infected with *M. avium* do not give a positive reaction. It is a more accurate test than the single I/D test and inflammatory responses is characterized by hot, painful and diffuse swelling.

4. Comparative test : This test depends on the greater sensitivity to homologous tuberculin and is carried out where the presence of Johne's disease or avian T.B. is suspected or skin T.B. is apparent. Avian and bovine tuberculin are injected simultaneously into two separate sites on the same side of the neck, 12 cm apart and one above the other and the test is read 72 h later. The greater the two reactions indicates the organism responsible for the sensitization. It is not generally recommended for primary use. It is recommended when a high incidence of avian T.B. or Johne's disease is anticipated or when vaccination against Johne's disease has been carried out. The comparative test is adequate to differentiate between vaccination against Johne's disease and tuberculosis.

Potency of tuberculins : For maximum specificity tuberculin (PPD) prepared from *M. bovis* is recommended. A dose between 5000 and 10,000 tuberculin units (0.1 ml tuberculin containing 0.1 or 0.2 mg of bovine PPD) is considered to be most suitable. For farmed deer a special tuberculin is used which contains 2 mg tuberculin/ml.

Desensitization : When a suspicious reactor is encountered, it is to be retested. However, it is complicated by the phenomenon of desensitization. After a SID test the period of desensitization is short and should not be retested before 60 days. However, after a stormont test desensitization may persist for as long as 6 months. If tuberculin is injected so that the test is made in the desensitized period no reaction will occur in infected animals.

Tuberculous cattle go through a period of desensitization immediately before and after calving and as many as 30% give false negative reaction returning to a positive status 4-6 weeks later. Calves drinking colostrum from infected dams give positive reactions for up to 3 weeks after birth even though they may not be infected.

Anergic animals are having lesions of TB but do not react to a cutaneous delayed hypersensitivity test. This can be overcome by injecting 0.2 mg tuberculin with reading at 48-72 h.

Summary of TB testing : it is usual to use the SID as a routine procedure. Annual testing of all cattle, quarantine of test positive herds and a movement ban into TB free areas has been effective in TB control schemes. Although sensitivity and specificity is high, false positive and false negative reactions occur.

False positive reaction (no gross reactors) : occurs in the following cases.

- Animal sensitized to other mycobacterial allergens, including those of human or avian tuberculosis or Johne's disease, relatively non-pathogenic mycobacteria eg. skin TB and ingestion of non pathogenic mycobacteria.
- Animals sensitized to other allergens eg., *N. farcinicus*.
- Reactors which are thought to be non-specific can be retested using whole blood IFN-γ assay 8-28 days after the skin test.

False negative reactions : occurs in the following cases.

(1) Advanced cases of T.B. (2) Early cases (< 6 weeks after infection) (3) Cow calves during preceding 6 weeks (4) Animals desensitized by tuberculin administration during the preceding 8-60 days (5) Old cattle (6) Low potency tuberculin or bacterial contamination of the tuberculin (7) Variable dose with multidose syringe.

Clinical examination and necropsy : Many cattle with bovine TB are clinically normal. Some cows with extensive miliary tuberculous lesions also appear clinically normal, but progressive emaciation unassociated with other signs should arouse suspicion of TB. Capricious appetite and fluctuating temperature are also commonly associated with the disease. Pulmonary involvement is eventually characterised by chronic cough, together with dyspnoea and other signs of low-grade pneumonia. Affected animals are docile and sluggish, but the eyes remain bright and alert.

Microscopy : M. bovis can be demonstrated microscopically on direct smears from clinical samples, and on prepared tissue materials. Tissue smears from affected organs stained by the Ziehl-Neelsen (ZN) method can be used to demonstrate the presence of acid-fast mycobacteria, red bacilli on a pale blue background (methylene blue staining), and appear on a green background if re-stained with malachite green. Examination of a haematoxylin-eosin-stained section of lesion for each case that is positive on smear is valuable. This technique is cheap, practical and a useful preliminary diagnostic step in developing countries where other laboratory facilities are not available; furthermore, identification in clinical samples and pathological specimens can be performed rapidly.

Culture on artificial media : Specimens are taken from affected lymph nodes and parenchymatous organs such as lungs, liver, spleen, etc. In animals with positive intradermal skin tests but showing no gross pathological lesions, samples from the retropharyngeal, bronchial, mediastinal and mesenteric lymph nodes are collected routinely for culture examination; the supramammary and mandibular glands and liver are sometimes included. Specimens are ground in silver sand, macerated or homogenised and decontaminated. Following centrifugation the sediment is often inoculated onto a set of solid media slopes consisting of egg-based media such as LJ, Coletsos base and Stonebrink's media. Slopes of these media containing pyruvate are inoculated, usually in duplicate, and an agar-based medium, such as Middlebrook 7H10 or 7H11, is also often used. Stonebrink's medium containing sodium pyruvate without glycerol is possibly the best medium. Colonies of *M. bovis* are expected to appear after 3–5 weeks of incubation at 37^0C.

Serological tests: CFT, FAT, direct bacterial agglutination, precipitin and haemagglutination tests have been developed but have little value for the routine diagnosis of T.B. ELISA which examines antibody to defined antigen but not crude as appear useful in detecting non-specific reactors. An in vitro assay of cell mediated reactivity by detection and quantitation of γ IFN known as IFN γ is licensed and commercially available in some countries. It is based on the detection of IFN γ liberated from WBC in whole blood cultutres incubated with PPD tuberculin. It can detect infected cattle earlier in infection than the skin test.

Molecular diagnostics : Culture is still internationally considered the gold standard for detection of mycobacteria; however, the intensity of labour required and the possible presence of viable non-cultivable mycobacteria in some clinical specimens requires more appropriate methods. Molecular diagnostic methods are in principle attractive replacements for traditional procedures, but such tests should have demonstrable, sustained improvement in sensitivity, specificity and reproducibility. They may be convenient and less costly when used for high throughput, but the availability of appropriate resources and trained staff is important and must be considered, particularly in developing countries. There is often a tendency to underestimate the difficulties inherent in introducing and applying these technologies to pathogens such as mycobacteria. In mycobacteriology, for obvious reasons, molecular technologies have been applied primarily to enhance detection and typing of *M. tuberculosis.* More recently, however, through international collaborative efforts, attention has been directed at *M. bovis* as a significant animal pathogen with zoonotic potential. The intracellular nature and impermeability of mycobacterial cell walls, together with the presence of polymerase chain reaction (PCR) inhibitors in clinical specimens, limit the efficiency of PCR detection. This can be problematic and impact on the potential uses of PCR detection with certain clinical specimens and in particular with specimens taken from tuberculous cattle, where low numbers of bacilli are common. Although amplification-based detection kits are commercially available, a recent review indicates that detection of *M. bovis* in animals has focused primarily on 'in house' amplification-based systems. Molecular biology techniques have now provided a means to detect and differentiate *M. bovis* isolates. Such differentiation should enable systematic epidemiological surveys to be conducted and, potentially, the origins of infection to be traced. Fingerprinting of *M. bovis* has been extremely effective using the restriction fragment analysis technique referred to as REA. However, widespread adoption of the method has been curtailed by issues such as potential cost and difficulties in technology transfer. A modified method of pulse field gel electrophoresis (PFGE) for *M. bovis* has had little uptake generally, as most methods now have advanced to exploiting the repetitive DNA sequences that occur in the mycobacterial genomes. Two types of repetitive DNA are known in bacterial genomes—dispersed repeats and tandem repeats. Dispersed repeats include mobile genetic elements, including insertion sequences (ISs) and prophages. Most of these ISs are located in the same genome position in members of the MTC; however, there are significant differences between species that are useful for diagnostics. The insertion element IS*6110*, which belongs to the IS3 family, is the most abundant and best-characterised. The IS*6110* copy number varies from 0 to 25 in MTC bacteria, whereas in *M. bovis* isolates the IS*6110* copy number is low, often occurring singly, especially in isolates from cattle. Interestingly, and usefully exploitable, the IS*6110* copy number is often higher in *M. bovis* isolates from more 'exotic' animal species. Molecular technologies are currently rarely employed in developing countries, and where they are available, priority is often given to human cases.

Treatment : T.B. in animals is treated in the same line as of human treatment. Drugs which are used in humans such as isoniazid, combinations of streptomycin and paraaminosalicylic and other acids have been used in animal with encouraging results. Isoniazid can be sued as prophylaxis and treatment. Isoniazid @ 5 mg/Kg BW for one and half months has been found beneficial against T.B. in cattle.

Control : Eradication of bovine T.B. has been virtually achieved in many countries with adoption of test and slaughter policy.

1. ***Control on a herd basis :*** It includes removal of infected animals, prevention of spread of infection and avoidance of further introduction of the disease.

a. Tuberculin testing : All the animals over 3 months of age should be tested by tuberculin test and positive animals should be disposed of according to local legislation. The comparative test should be used where infection with *M. paratuberculosis* or *M. avium* is anticipated. Retesting of the herd should be carried out at 3 months intervals until a negative test is obtained. A further test is conducted 6 months later and if found negative it may be classed as free of the disease. Subsequent tests should be carried out annually.

b. Prevention of spread :

- Hygienic measures such as cleaning of feed or water troughs thoroughly.
- Calves should be fed tuberculosis free or pasteurized milk.
- Farm attendants should be checked as they provide a source of infection.

2. Control on an area basis

a. *Education :* Livestock owners must be apprized of the economic and public health significance of the disease, its manifestation and necessity for the various steps in the eradication program.

b. *Vaccination :* BCG vaccination is the only method available for field use. Vaccination must be repeated annually and the vaccinated animal remains positive to the tuberculin test. The vaccine is not so effective and immunity is not strong. It is used as a temporary measure when the incidence of T.B. is high.

There are a number of newer prospective vaccines including subunit and synthetic peptide vaccine, attenuated mutant of *M. bovis* and antigens expressed in attenuated live vaccine vectors. It is also possible to differentiate infected from vaccinated animals.

Problem of eradication : Complete eradication of T.B. has not really been achieved in any country. Although a state of virtual eradication has been in existence for years but minor recrudescence occur. The major problems arise are as follows.

- No visible lesion (NVL) reactors : The percentage of reactors with NVL at slaughter rises steeply as the disease prevalence decreases.

- Breakdown : Individual herds with no positive animals may have disease again because an anergic carrier has been left in the herd.
- Large herd : Another kind of difficulty in eradication is where cattle are run under very extensive conditions on large ranches or stations.
- Wildlife reservoirs : The spread of disease from badger and deer to cattle in U.K. and brush tailed possum in New Zealand is a major problem.
- Control of T.B. in pigs : *M. bovis* infection in pigs usually result from the feeding of infected milk, skim milk or whey to pigs, allowing cattle and pigs to graze the same pasture. The first step in the control of T.B. in a pig herd is to remove the source of infection and then to test and remove the reacting animals which is not an efficient method.

Further reading

Dorman, S.E. and Chaisson, R.E. (2007). From magic bullets back to the magic mountain: the rise of extensively drug-resistant tuberculosis. *Nat. Med.* 13: 295–298.

Dye, C. (2006). Targets for global tuberculosis control. *Int. J. Tuberc. Lung Dis.* 10 : 460–462.

Dye, C. (2009). Doomsday postponed? Preventing and reversing epidemics of drug-resistant tuberculosis. *Nat. Rev. Microbiol.* 7: 81–87.

Dye, C., Hosseini, M. and Watt, C. (2007). Did we reach the 2005 targets for tuberculosis control? *Bull W.H.O.* 85: 364–369.

Dye, C., Watt, C.J. and Bleed, D.M. (2005). Evolution of tuberculosis control and prospects for reducing tuberculosis incidence, prevalence and deaths globally. *JAMA.* 293: 2767–2775.

Epidemiology and Challenges of Global TB (2010). CID 50 (Suppl 3): S163

Frieden, T.R. (2009). Lessons from tuberculosis control for public health. *Int. J. Tuberc. Lung Dis.* 13: 421–428.

Gillespie, S.H. (2002). Evolution of drug resistance in *Mycobacterium tuberculosis:* clinical and molecular perspective. *Antimicrob Agents Chemother.* 46: 267–274.

Hopewell, P.C., Pai, M., Maher, D., Uplekar, M. and Raviglione, M.C. (2006). International standards for tuberculosis care. *Lancet Infect. Dis.* 6: 710–725.

Jassal, M. and Bishai, W.R. (2009). Extensively drug resistant tuberculosis. *Lancet Infect. Dis.* 9:19–30.

Jensen, P.A., Lambert, L.A., Iademarco, M.F. and Ridzon, F. (2005). Centers for Diseases Control and Prevention. Guideline for preventing the transmission of *Mycobacterium tuberculosis* in health-care settings. *MMWR Recomm. Rep.* 54 : 1–141.

Khatri, G.R. and Frieden, T. R. (2000). The status and prospects of tuberculosis control in India. *Int. J Tuberc. Lung Dis.* 4: 193–200.

Khatri, G.R. and Frieden, T. R. (2002). Controlling tuberculosis in India. *N. Engl. J. Med.* 347: 1420–1425.

Lonroth, K. and Raviglione, M. (2008). Global epidemiology of tuberculosis: Prospects for control. *Semin. Respir. Crit. Care Med.* 29: 481–491.

Maher, D., Dyee, C., Floyd, K. (2007). Planning to improve global health: the next decade of tuberculosis control. *Bull W.H.O.* 85: 341–347.

Marmot, M. G. and Bell, R.(2009).How will the financial crisis affect health? *BMJ.* 338: b1314.

Mukherjee, J.S., Rich, M.L. and Socci, A.R. (2004). Programmes and principles in treatment of multidrug-resistant tuberculosis. *Lancet.* 363: 474–481.

Prasad, R., Nautiyal, R. G., Mukherji, P. K., Jain, A., Singh, K. and Ahuja, R. C. (2003). Diagnostic evaluation of pulmonary tuberculosis: what do doctors of modern medicine do in India? *Int.J. Tuberc. Lung Dis.* 7: 52–57.

Prasad, R., Nautiyal, R. G., Mukherji, P. K., Jain, A., Singh, K. and Ahuja, R C. (2002). Treatment of new pulmonary tuberculosis patients: what do allopathic doctors do in India? Int. *J. Tuberc. Lung Dis.* 6: 895–902.

Ranjbhandary, S.S., Marks, S.M. and Bock, N.N. (2004). Costs of patients hospitalized for multidrug-resistant tuberculosis. *Int. J. Tuberc. Lung Dis.* 8: 1012–1016.

Raviglione, M.C. and Pio, A. (2002). Evolution of WHO policies for tuberculosis control, 1948–2001. *Lancet.* 359: 775–780.

Raviglione, M.C. (2007). The new Stop TB Strategy and the Global Plan to Stop TB, 2006–2015. *Bull W.H.O.* 85: 327.

The Global Plan to Stop TB. 2006–2015: actions for life towards a world free of tuberculosis. Geneva: World Health Organization.

Tupasi, T.E., Gupta, R. and Quelapio, M.I. (2006). Feasibility and cost-effectiveness of treating multidrug-resistant tuberculosis: a cohort study in the Philippines. *PLoS Med.*3: e352.

World Health Organization (2006). Global tuberculosis: surveillance, planning, financing. Geneva: World Health Organization.

World Health Organization (2008). Global Tuberculosis Control, Geneva.

World Health Organization (2009). Global Tuberculosis Control, Geneva.

Young, D.B., Perkins, M.D., Duncan, K. and Barry, C.E. (2008). Confronting the scientific obstacles to global control of tuberculosis. *J. Clin. Invest.* 118: 1255–1265.

13

Brucellosis

Synonyms : Bang's disease, Contagious abortion, Infectious abortion, Enzootic abortion, Undulant fever, Malta fever, Mediterranean fever

Brucellosis, one of the most ancient diseases, continues to be a problem for humans and animals throughout the world causing enormous economic losses and significant human morbidity in endemic areas. The bacterial pathogen is classified by the CDC as a category B pathogen that has the potential for development as a bioweapon. It is one of the important zoonotic disease and considered as the most common laboratory acquired pathogen with >5 lakh human cases reported annually around the world. Brucellosis is a chronic infection which can result in infertility, delayed heat, interrupted lactation, loss of calves, wool, meat and milk production in animals and undulant fever in humans. Although in most of the countries, brucellosis is a nationally notifiable disease and reportable to the local health authority, it is underreported and official numbers constitute only a fraction of true incidence of the disease. Although the true incidence of human brucellosis is unknown, the estimated burden of the disease varies widely from <0.03 to >160 per 1 lakh population. Although only 17 countries in the world are free from the disease, it has been reported in many countries including India. Bovine brucellosis is endemic in all the states in India and appears to be on the increase in recent time, perhaps due to increased trade and rapid movement of livestock. The preponderance of natural bull service in rural India is perhaps yet another important factor in the maintenance and spread of infection. The Government of India has made it mandatory to regularly screen all the breeding bulls from artificial insemination centres, for brucellosis and to use brucellosis free bulls for semen production.

Etiology : *Brucella sp.* are facultative intracellular Gram – ve coccobacilli, nonspore forming and non-capsulated. It infects macrophages with principal involvement of liver, spleen and bone marrow. Nine *Brucella species* are currently recognized, seven of them that affect terrestrial animals are : *B. abortus, B. melitensis, B. suis, B. ovis, B. canis, B.*

neotomae and *B. microti* and two that affect marine mammals are *B. ceti* and *B. pinnipedialis.* The first three species are called classical Brucella and within these species seven biovars are recognized for *B. abortus,* three for *B. melitensis* and five for *B. suis*. The remaining species have not been differentiated into biovars.

Brucella spp. are facultative intracellular Gram negative coccobacilli, nonmotile, non-spore forming and non-capsulated. With the advent of molecular techniques and the discovery of new species, the following system is currently in use. *Brucella cetaceae, Brucella melitensis* subdivided into *Brucella melitensis* biovar *Abortus, Brucella melitensis* biovar *Canis, Brucella melitensis* biovar *Melitensis, Brucella melitensis* biovar *Neotomae, Brucella melitensis* biovar *Ovis, Brucella melitensis* biovar *Suis* and *Brucella pinnipediae*. The main pathogenic species worldwide are *B. melitensis* responsible for ovine and caprine brucellosis and producing the most severe infections in humans ; *B. abortus* the main etiologic agent of bovine brucellosis, *B. suis* responsible for swine brucellosis. These 3 species may cause abortion and infertility in their hosts causing huge economic losses. *B. ovis* and *B. canis* are responsible for ram epididymitis and canine brucellosis respectively. The *B. melitensis*, *B. abortus* and *B. suis* contain several biovars. Species and biovars are currently distinguished by differential tests based on phenotypic characterization by serotyping, phage typing, dye sensitivity, CO_2 requirement, H_2S production and metabolic properties. Several brucella strains have also been isolated from marine mammalian species such as seal, dolphin, porpoise, whale and otter species. The most pathogenic and invasive species is *B. melitensis* followed by in descending order *B. suis*, *B. abortus* and *B. canis*. *B. melitensis* is the principal cause of human brucellosis worldwide and may accounts for up to 90% of all brucellosis cases with *B. melitensis* type 1 predominant in India and Spain, type 2 in northwestern Greece and type 3 in turkey.

Brucella melitensis, *B. abortus*, and *B. suis* strains may occur either as smooth (S) or rough (R) strains expressing smooth LPS (S-LPS) containing O chain or rough LPS (R-LPS) lacking O chain as major surface antigen respectively. The *B. ovis* and *B. canis* are two naturally R species expressing thus R-LPS as major surface antigen. S-LPS has been shown to be a major virulence factor. Its O chain moiety represents the most exposed antigenic structure of the Brucella cell surface and an immunodominant antigen in antibody responses of the infected host as well as involved in serological reactions in sero-diagnosis of infections caused by smooth Brucella strains. Besides LPS, the outer membrane of Brucella is mainly composed of major outer membrane proteins (OMPs) which have potential as protective antigens.

Epidemiology : The geographical distribution of brucellosis is constantly changing with new foci emerging or reemerging. The disease is endemic in many countries of the world with the exception of few countries where bovine brucellosis has been eradicated or not reported. These countries are Australia,

Canada, Cyprus, Denmark, Finland, The Netherlands, New Zealand, Norway, Sweden and the United Kingdom (excluding Northern Ireland), Germany, Belgium, Luxembourg, Switzerland, France and Austria. In India bovine brucellosis is endemic in all the states of the countries. Besides, seropositivity to brucellosis has been reported in other species of animals viz., buffalo, mithuns, yaks, sheep, goat, swine, equine, camel, dog, poultry, wild animals as well as in human beings. Consumption of unpasteurized milk and their products especially soft cheese, yoghurts and ice-cream, undercooked traditional delicacies such as liver and spleen are mainly responsible for human brucellosis. Further, contact with vaginal discharge, urine, faeces and blood of infected animals through broken skin and mucous membrane of conjunctiva and inhalation of the organism can cause the disease. The disease is an occupational hazard for livestock owners, abattoir workers, dairy workers, shepherds, farmers, veterinarians and laboratory workers. An estimated 5 lakhs human infections per year still occur worldwide. Among animals, the predominant route of exposure for smooth strains of Brucella is through ingestion or inhalation of organisms that are present in fetal fluids or other birth products.

Global distribution and economic impact : The geographical distribution of brucellosis is constantly changing, with new foci emerging or reemerging. The epidemiology of human brucellosis has drastically changed over the past few years because of various sanitary, socioeconomic and political reasons, together with increased international travel. The disease occurs worldwide, except in those countries where bovine brucellosis *(B. abortus)* has been eradicated or not reported during last 5 years. These countries include Australia, Canada, Cyprus, Denmark, Finland, The Netherlands, New Zealand, Norway, Sweden and the United Kingdom (excluding Northern Ireland), Germany, Belgium, Luxembourg, Switzerland, France and Austria.

Zoonoses : Five out of the nine known Brucella species can infect humans and the most pathogenic and invasive species for humans is *B. melitensis*, followed in descending order by *B. suis*, *B. abortus* and *B. canis*. *B. ceti* (marine brucellae) is also transmissible to human beings. *B. melitensis, B. suis* and *B. abortus* are highly infectious and readily aerosolized and listed as potential bio-weapons by the Centers for Disease Control and Prevention in the USA. The symptoms of brucellosis are easily confused with influenza, enteric fever, rheumatic fever etc. In endemic areas, humans can get infected via contact with infected animals or consumption of their products, mostly milk and milk products especially cheese made from unpasteurized milk of sheep and goats and rennet from infected lambs and kids. Farm workers, veterinarians, ranchers and meat packing employees are considered at higher risk. *B. abortus* and *B. suis* infections usually affect occupational groups while *B. melitensis* infections occur more frequently than the other Brucella species in the general population. Consumption of sheep or goat milk containing *B. melitensis* is an important source of human brucellosis worldwide and has caused several outbreaks (99%). In countries where milk and dairy products are always pasteurized before consumption, brucellosis principally affect persons who are in close contact with animals and animal products. Although Brucella is considered highly infectious when encountered via the respiratory route (e.g. 10 bacteria required for infection in mice), inhalation of Brucella is not a common route of infection.

Human brucellosis : The incubation period of brucellosis normally is 1-3 weeks. But it can be several months before showing signs of infection. *B. melitensis* is associated with acute infection whereas the infections with other species are usually subacute and prolonged. Most common symptoms of brucellosis include undulant fever in which the temperature can vary from 37° C in the morning to 40° C in the afternoon, night sweats with peculiar odor, chills and weakness. Common symptoms also include malaise, insomnia, anorexia, headache, arthralgia, constipation, sexual impotence, nervousness and depression. It affects many internal organs and diverse symptoms include encephalitis, meningitis, spondylitis, arthritis, endocarditis, orchitis and prostatitis. Spontaneous abortions, mostly in the first and second trimesters of pregnancy are seen in pregnant women infected with Brucella. Although Brucella endocarditis is of rare occurrence (<2%) , it is commonly associated with *B. melitensis* infection and accounts for at least 80% of deaths due to brucellosis. The symptoms and signs of brucellosis may be confused with enteric fever, malaria, rheumatic fever, tuberculosis, cholecystitis, thrombophlebitis, fungal infection, autoimmune disease and tumors. Live animal vaccines *B. melitensis* Rev. 1 and *B. abortus* strain 19 are known to cause disease in humans. The course of disease with vaccine strains is shorter and more benign.

Animal brucellosis : The most frequent clinical sign following infection with Brucella is abortion. The principal strain that infects cattle is *B. abortus*. However, cattle can also become transiently infected by *B. suis* and more commonly by *B. melitensis* when they share pasture with infected pigs, goats and sheep. *B. melitensis* and *B. suis* can be transmitted by cow's milk and cause a serious public health threat. The profound manifestation in pregnant females is abortion usually in the second half of gestation with retention of placenta and metritis. There is 25% reduction in milk production in infected cows. The brucellae localize in the supra-mammary lymph nodes and mammary glands of 80% of the infected animals and thus continue to secrete the pathogen in milk throughout their lives. Most of the cows abort only once although the placenta will be heavily infected at subsequent apparently normal calvings.

The main etiologic agent of brucellosis in goats is *B. melitensis* although it can be infected with *B. abortus*. Like cattle, brucellosis in goats is characterized by late abortion, still births, decreased fertility and low milk production. Sheep brucellosis can be divided into classical brucellosis and ram epididymitis. Ram epididymitis is caused by non-zoonotic *B. ovis*, whereas classical brucellosis is caused by *B. melitensis* and constitutes a major public health threat similar to goat brucellosis. Swine brucellosis is characterized by abortion, orchitis, lameness, hind limb paralysis, spondylitis and metritis. Camels can be infected by *B. abortus* and *B. melitensis* when they are grazed in the same pasture with infected sheep, goat and cattle. The causative agent of canine brucellosis is *B. canis* but sporadic cases due to *B. abortus*, *B. suis* and *B. melitensis* have been reported.

Diagnosis : Human brucellosis can be confused with a number disease conditions. Accurate and fast diagnosis of human brucellosis is very important as delay or misdiagnosis usually results in treatment failures, relapses, chronic courses, and high case fatality rate. Isolation of Brucella from blood, bone marrow, lymph nodes or cerebrospinal fluids remains the gold standard for diagnosis of brucellosis in humans. The cultural isolation has disadvantages such as slow growth and poor sensitivity. *B. melitensis* is more readily cultured from clinical samples than *B. abortus*.

Serological tests for antibody detection that measure the ability of serum to agglutinate a standardized amount of killed *B. abortus* reflect the presence of antibody against O-side chain derived from lipopolysaccharide. Brucella specific IgM appearing at the end of the first week of the disease followed by IgG are still the most common and useful measures for the laboratory diagnosis of brucellosis. These agglutinations tests, however, are not useful for diagnosis of infection caused by *B. canis* (a naturally O- side chain deficient strain). Serum agglutination test known as standard tube agglutination test (STAT) is commonly used for diagnosis of acute brucellosis whereas 2-mercaptoethanol (2 ME) and complement tests (CFT) are used for chronic brucellosis. 2ME that disrupts disulfide bonds making IgM inactive and permitting only Brucella agglutination by IgG resistant to 2ME. Other useful tests for diagnosis of human brucellosis are the Rose Bengal test (RBT), CIE, Coombs test, immunocapture agglutination test, latex agglutination and indirect ELISA. Molecular test like PCR has been found to be a useful and more sensitive tool for diagnosis of brucellosis. Brucellosis in cattle is diagnosed from pooled milk samples by Brucella ring test and blood samples by slide agglutination test and STAT. For ovine and caprine brucellosis the Rose Bengal plate agglutination, CF and indirect ELISA are usually recommended.

Treatment : The ideal treatment for brucellosis is a combination of two antibiotics since therapy with single antibiotic has been associated with high relapse rates. The combination of doxycycline with streptomycin (DS) is currently the best therapeutic option with less side effects and less relapses especially in cases of acute and localized forms of brucellosis. Neither doxycycline nor streptomycin alone can prevent multiplication of intracellular brucellae. The disadvantage of the combination therapy is that streptomycin must be administered parenterally for 3 weeks. A combination of doxycycline (6 weeks) with parenterally administered gentamycin (5mg/kg) for 7 days is considered an acceptable alternate regimen. However, WHO has changed the recommendation for treatment of adult brucellosis to doxycycline (200 mg/day orally) and rifampicin(600-900 mg/day orally)(DR.). However DS therapy is more effective than DR therapy.

Vaccines : Besides the public health concern, brucellosis in animals have an economic impact as they cause infertility, reduce milk production and infertility. In endemic areas with high prevalence of disease, the only way of controlling and eradicating the disease is by vaccination of susceptible animals and culling of infected animals. The most commonly used vaccines against bovine brucellosis are *B. abortus* strain 19 and the recently USDA approved strain RB51. The latter one unlike strain 19 does not interfere with the serological testing. The persistence of antibodies to *B. abortus* strain 19 vaccine depends on the age of the animals vaccinated. *B. melitensis* strain Rev 1 although highly infectious to human, is considered to be the best vaccine available for the control of ovine and caprine brucellosis administered by conjunctival route. Again, it can not be used in pregnant animals as it causes abortion. However, vaccinated animals can not be differentiated from the infected animals using these vaccines. The new live attenuated rough *B. melitensis* vaccines which are devoid of the O side chain are in the process of development. Live human vaccines *B. abortus* strain 19-BA and strain 104M are being used only the former Soviet Union and China. However, brucellosis in animals can only be controlled by vaccination along with good management practices and zoosanitary measures.

There are a number of vaccines available for use in animals against brucellosis.

1) ***B. abortus* strain 19 (Live attenuated) :** It is the most acceptable and widely used vaccine to prevent bovine brucellosis due to its relative safety, potency and practicality of production and convenience of use in cattle. It differs from *B. abortus* biovar 1 strain in its requirement for CO2 and sensitivity to thionine blue, penicillin and safranin. It is the only *Brucella sp.* strain that is inhibited by erythritol. It was isolated from the milk of a Jersey cow as a virulent strain in 1923. It had been attenuated after keeping in the laboratory at room temperature for over a year. It is having smooth morphology. Although it is of low virulence for cattle, vaccination of pregnant cows can result abortions in 1 to 2.5% cases under field conditions and orchitis in bulls. It is also pathogenic for human beings. Further, the presence of LPS with an O chain on strain 19 explains the appearance and persistence of antibodies in serum following administration of this vaccine. These antibodies are detected in the serological assays used for the diagnosis of brucellosis and are the major problem associated with strain 19 vaccination since they prevent easy differentiation of vaccinated from infected cattle. The appearance and persistence of these antibodies depends on age, dose and route of vaccination. It is usually given at 4 to 8 months of age. Vaccination with it is not curative and vaccination will not cure the infected animals. It does not induce absolute

immunity but increases resistance to *B. abortus*. It is only 70% effective against field challenge by preventing unrestricted multiplication of *B. abortus* in the uterus and mammary gland. Lyophilised vaccine should be used within 3 hours of reconstitution. The dose of strain 19 vaccine administered S/C to heifer calves at 4 to 8 months of age contains $5X10^{10}$ viable Brucella cells. The vaccination of heifers practically eliminates the occurrence of abortions in a herd. When 80% female population has been vaccinated, there is gradual decline in prevalence of bovine brucellosis. Administration of strain 19 vaccine into the conjunctival sac (1 to 2 doses of $5\text{-}10X10^{10}$ at 4 and 8 months of age) results in good protection. In the event of an outbreak, the vaccination of adult cattle with strain 19 vaccine may be advantageous, particularly in large dairy herds and the herds where a large proportions of animals have not been previously been vaccinated. Mature cows inoculated with a $3\text{-}10X10^{8}$ organisms/dose are protected for at least 12 months. Because it has also been found in the semen of vaccinated bulls, its use in males has been restricted or prohibited. Uni or bilateral hygromas especially of the carpal joints may occasionally follow inoculation of heifers with strain 19 vaccine. A progressive, erosive, non-suppurative arthritis of the stifle joints has been reported in young cattle in brucellosis free herds that had been vaccinated with strain 19 vaccine. There is rise of temperature ranging from 40.5 to 42°C lasting for 2-3 days. There is no evidence of the spread of strain 19 to unvaccinated cattle although it can be excreted in milk for 2-3 months in vaccinated cows after calving or abortion. The infection of human consuming milk of vaccinated animals has not been reported but undulant fever in human accidentally infected with the vaccine has been reported. When eradication is the aim, vaccination should be stopped once the incidence falls below 0.2% and infected animals are eliminated.

2) ***B. melitensis* Rev 1 (Live attenuated) :** Rev 1 vaccine is a live attenuated *B. melitensis* smooth strain derived from a virulent *B. melitensis* isolate which became dependent on streptomycin for its growth. It provides protection against infection to *B. melitensis* in sheep and goats as well as infection with *B. ovis*. Although it is attenuated, it retains some virulency and causes abortion if it is used in pregnancy. In rams, it is avirulent. In cattle, it may sometimes give better protection than strain 19.

3) ***B. abortus* strain 45/20 (Inactivated) :** The persistence of serum antibodies following strain 19 vaccination interfered with serological testing. The use of a live attenuated rough strain could avoid this problem if the strain is stable and confer solid protective immunity. *B. abortus* smooth strain 45/0 was isolated from a cow in 1922 and a rough derivative was obtained after 20 passages in guinea pigs called strain 45/20. It was able to protect guinea pigs and cattle from brucella infection. However, when used as a live vaccine, strain 45/20 was not stable and tended to revert to the smooth, virulent form. In order to overcome the lack of stability of the live strain 45/20 vaccine, it was used as bacterin incorporated in water in oil adjuvant. Protection induced by

two doses has been found to be superior to strain 19 and it may not induce diagnostically undesirable antibodies or abortions. However, the variability of reported protection and the occurrence of severe local reactions at the site of vaccine injection in some animals eventually prompted the discontinuation of strain 45/20 vaccination.

4) ***B. abortus*** **RB 51 (Live attenuated) :** In order to avoid the diagnostic problems with smooth strains, the search for rough strains devoid of O chain, stable and sufficiently attenuated as vaccine candidate was started. The fact that *B. abortus* strain 45/20, a rough organism while little or no ability to induce O chain antibodies could induce significant protection against infection with *B. abortus* indicated that rough organisms can be used to induce protective immune responses while avoiding the diagnostic problems. Such a derivative was produced from a rifampicin resistant mutant of *B. abortus* strain 2308 called *Brucella abortus* strain RB51. R stands for rough and B stands for Brucella. It is devoid of O chain and roughness is stable after multiple passages *in vivo* and *in vitro* through various species of animals. Due to absence of O chain it does not usually induce O chain antibodies measurable by serological tests used in the diagnosis of brucellosis regardless of age, dose or frequency of injection. It can be used both in high and low brucellosis prevalence area and immunity is at least 1 year similar to or better than immunity induced by strain 19. The dose is 1-3.4 X 10^{10} S/C and age of vaccination is 4 months. Pregnant animals can safely be vaccinated S/C with 10^{9} RB51 organisms without the induction of abortions or placentitis. Intravenous inoculations of pregnant cattle with 10^{10} organisms lead to placental and fetal infections but not to abortion. The protective immunity induced by strain RB51 is solely T cell mediated. It is able to protect against infections with *B. abortus, B. melitensis, B. suis* and *B. ovis*. All species of vaccinated animals were serologically negative to all conventional serological tests for brucellosis.

5) BS2 vaccine (Live attenuated) : A smooth strain of *B. suis* biovar 1 has been in use as an oral vaccine to control brucellosis in cattle, sheep, goat and pigs in China since 1971. It protects cattle, against *B. abortus*, is safe if administered orally and does not induce persistent antibody titres. Although it has been widely used in China, it is not recommended by OIE.

Further reading

Adone, R., Francia, M. and Ciuchini, F. (2008). Evaluation of *Brucella melitensis* B115 as rough-phenotype vaccine against *B. melitensis* and *B. ovis* infections. *Vaccine.* 26 : 4913–4917.

Al Dahouk, S., Tomaso, H., Nockler, K., Neubauer, H. and Frangoulidis, D. (2003). Laboratory-based diagnosis of brucellosis - a review of the literature. Part I: Techniques for direct detection and identification of *Brucella* spp. *Clin. Lab.* 49 : 487-505.

Al Dahouk, S., Tomaso, H., Nockler, K., Neubauer, H. and Frangoulidis, D. (2003). Laboratory-based diagnosis of brucellosis - a review of the literature. Part II: serological tests for brucellosis. *Clin. Lab.* 49 : 577-89.

Arroyo, I., Carrera, M.J., Lopez Rodriguez, A.M., Sapina, A., Lafuente, Lopez. and Sacristan, A.R. (2006). Probable transmission of brucellosis by breast milk. *J. Trop. Pediatr.* 52 : 380–381.

Barbuddhe, S.B., Kumar, P., Malika, S.V., Singh, D.K. and Gupta, L.K. (2000). Seropositivity for intracellular bacterial infections among abattoir associated personnels. *J. Commun. Dis.* 32 : 295-9.

Bayindir, Y., Sonmez, E., Aladag, A. and Buyukberber, N. (2003). Comparison of five antimicrobial regimens for the treatment of brucellar spondylitis: a prospective, randomized study. *J. Chemother.* 15 : 466-71.

Bikas, C., Jelastopulu, E., Leotsinidis, M. and Kondakis, X. (2003). Epidemiology of human brucellosis in a rural area of northwestern Peloponnese in Greece. *Eur. J. Epidemiol.* 18 : 267-74.

Boschirali, M.L., Foulongue, V. and Callaghan, D. (2001). Brucellosis: a worldwide zoonosis. *Curr. Opin. Microbiol.* 4 : 658-64.

Chakraborty, M., Patgiri, G.P. and Barman, N.N. (2000). Application of delayed-type hypersensitivity test (DTH) for the diagnosis of bovine brucellosis. *Indian Vet. J.* **77** : 924-5.

Corbel, M.J. (2002). Brucellosis: an overview. *Emerg. Infect. Dis.* 3 : 213-21.

Dahouk, S.A., Neubauer, H., Hensel, A., Schoneberg, I., Nockler, K., Alpers, K., Merzenich, H., Stark, K. and Jansen, A. (2007). Changing epidemiology of human brucellosis, Germany, 1962–2005. *Emerg. Infect. Dis.* 13 : 1895–1900.

DelVecchio, V.G., Kapatral, V., Redkar, R.J., Patra, G., Mujer, C. and Los, T. (2002). The genome sequence of the facultative intracellular pathogen *Brucella melitensis*. *Proc. Natl. Acad. Sci.* 99 : 443-8.

DelVecchio, V.G., Kapatral, V., Elzer, P., Patra, G., Mujer, C.V. (2002). The genome of *Brucella melitensis*. *Vet. Microbiol.* 90 : 587-92.

Dokuzoguz, B., Ergonul, O., Baykam, N., Esener, H., Kilic, S. and Celikbas, A. (2005). Characteristics of *B. melitensis* versus *B. abortus* bacteraemias. *J. Infect.* 50 : 41-5.

El Miedany, Y.M., El Gaafary, M., Baddour, M. and Ahmed, I. (2003). Human brucellosis: do we need to revise our therapeutic policy? *J. Rheumatol.* 30 : 2666-72.

Ergonul, O., Willke, A., Azap, A. and Tekeli, E. (2005). Revised definition of 'fever of unknown origin': limitations and opportunities. *J. Infect.* 50 : 1-5.

Ersoy, Y., Sonmez, E., Tevfik M.R. and But, A.D. (2005). Comparison of three different combination therapies in the treatment of human brucellosis. *Trop. Doct.* 35 : 210–212.

Falagas, M.E. and Bliziotis, I.A. (2006). Quinolones for treatment of human brucellosis: critical review of the evidence from microbiological and clinical studies. *Antimicrob. Agents Chemother.* 50 : 22–33.

Ficht, T.A. (2003). Intracellular survival of *Brucella*: defining the link with persistence. *Vet. Microbiol.* 92 : 213-23.

Garin-Bastuji, B., Blasco, J.M., Grayon, M. and Verger, J.M. (1998). *Brucella melitensis* infection in sheep: present and future. *Vet. Res.* 29 : 255–274.

Gorvel, J.P. and Moreno, E. (2002). Brucella intracellular life: from invasion to intracellular replication. *Vet. Microbiol.* 90 : 281-97.

Halling, S.M., Peterson-Burch, B.D., Bricker, B.J., Zuerner, R.L., Qing, Z. and Li, L.L. (2005). Completion of the genome sequence of *Brucella abortus* and comparison to the highly similar genomes of *Brucella melitensis* and *Brucella suis*. *J. Bacteriol.* 187 : 2715–2726.

Hamdy, M.E. and Amin, A.S. (2002). Detection of *Brucella* species in the milk of infected cattle, sheep, goats and camels by PCR. *Vet. J.* 163 : 299–305.

Hasanjani Roushan, M.R., Mohrez, M., Smailnejad Gangi, S.M., Soleimani-Amiri, M.J. and Hajiahmadi, M. (2004). Epidemiological features and clinical manifestations in 469 adult patients with brucellosis in Babol, Northern Iran. *Epidemiol. Infect.* 132 : 1109-14.

Irmak, H., Buzgan, T., Evirgen, O., Akdeniz, H., Demiroz, A.P. and Abdoel, T.H. (2004). Use of the *Brucella* IgM and IgG flow assays in the serodiagnosis of human brucellosis in an area endemic for brucellosis. *Am. J. Trop. Med. Hyg.* 70 : 688-94.

Isloor, S., Renukaradhya, G.J. and Rajasekhar, M. (1998). A serological survey of bovine brucellosis in India. *Rev. Sci. Tech.* 17 : 781-5.

Joshi, P.A., Kulkarni, R.D. and Powar, R.M. (2005). Modified cold Z-N staining for presumptive identification of Brucella. *Indian J. Med. Res.* 121 : 108-10.

Kadri, S.M., Rukhsana, A., Laharwal, M.A. and Tanvir, M. (2000). Seroprevalence of brucellosis in Kashmir (India) among patients with pyrexia of unknown origin. *J. Indian Med. Assoc.* 98 : 170-1.

Kattar, M.M., Zalloua, P.A., Araj, G.F. and Samaha-Kfoury, J. (2007). Development and evaluation of real-time polymerase chain reaction assays on whole blood and paraffin-embedded tissues for rapid diagnosis of human brucellosis. *Diagn. Microbiol. Infect. Dis.* 59 : 23–32.

Kochar, D.K., Sharma, B.V., Gupta, S., Jain, R., Gauri, L.A. and Srivastava, T. (2003). Pulmonary manifestations in brucellosis: a report on seven cases from Bikaner (north-west India). *J Assoc. Physicians India.* 51 : 33-6.

Kumar, P., Singh, D.K. and Barbuddhe, S.B. (1997). Serological evidence of brucellosis in sheep and goats. *Indian J. Anim. Sci.* 67 : 180-2.

Lapaque, N., Moriyon, I., Moreno, E. and Gorvel, J.P. (2005). Brucella lipopolysaccharide acts as a virulence factor. *Curr. Opin. Microbiol.* 8 : 60-6.

Mantur, B.G., Akki, A.S., Mangalgi, S.S., Patil, S.V., Gobbur, R.H. and Peerapur, B.V. (2004). Childhood brucellosis - a microbiological, epidemiological and clinical study. *J. Trop. Pediatr.* 50 : 153-7.

Mantur, B.G., Amarnath, S.K. and Shinde, R.S. (2007). Review of clinical and laboratory features of human brucellosis. *Indian J. Med. Microbiol.* 25 : 188–202.

Massis, F. De., Girolamo, A. Di., Petrini, A., Pizzigallo, E. and Giovannini, A. (2005). Correlation between animal and human brucellosis in Italy during the period 1997–2002. *Clin. Microbiol. Infect.* 11 : 632–636.

Mehra, K.N., Dhanesar, N.S. and Chaturvedi, V.K. (2000). Sero-prevalence of brucellosis in bovine in Madhya Pradesh. *Indian Vet. J.* 77 : 571-3.

Memish, Z., Mah, M.W., Al Mahmoud, S., Al Shaalan, M. and Khan, M.Y. (2000). Brucella bacteraemia: clinical and laboratory observations in 160 patients. *J. Infect.* 40 : 59-63.

Minas, A., Minas, M., Stournara, A. and Tselepidis, S. (2004). The "effects"of Rev-1 vaccination of sheep and goats on human brucellosis in Greece. *Prev. Vet. Med.* 64 : 41-7.

Moriyon, I., Grillo, M.J., Monreal, D. and Gonzalez, D. (2004). Rough vaccines in animal brucellosis: structural and genetic basis and present status. *Vet. Res.* 35 : 1–38.

Moriyon, I., Grillo, M.J., Monreal, D., Gonzalez, D., Marin, C. and Lopez-Goni, I. (2004). Rough vaccines in animal brucellosis: structural and genetic basis and present status. *Vet Res.* 35 : 1-38.

Mrunalini, N., Rama, S.P., Pandarinath, G.N. and Ramakrishna, R.M. (2000). Control of brucellosis in goats in a farm. *Indian Vet. J.* 77 : 932-5.

Munoz, P.M., Marin, C.M., Morreal, D., Gonzales, D., Garin-Bastuji, B. and Diaz, R. (2005). Efficacy of several serological tests and antigens for diagnosis of bovine brucellosis in the presence of false-positive serological results due to *Yersinia enterocolitica* O:9. *Clin. Diag. Lab. Immunol.* 12 : 141-51.

Orduna, A., Almaraz, A., Prado, A. and Gutierrez, M.P. (2000). Evaluation of an immunocapture-agglutination test (Brucellacapt) for serodiagnosis of human brucellosis. *J. Clin. Microbiol.* 38 : 4000–4005.

Palanduz, A., Palanduz, S., Guler, K. and Guler, N. (2000). Brucellosis in a mother and her young infant: probable transmission by breast milk. *Int. J. Infect. Dis.* 4 : 55-6.

Pappas, G., Panagopoulou, P., Christou, L. and Akritidis, N. (2006). *Brucella* as a biological weapon. *Cell Mol. Life Sci.* 63 : 2229–2236.

Pappas, G., Akritidis, N. and Tsianos, E. (2005). Effective treatments in the management of brucellosis. *Expert Opin. Pharmacother.* 6 : 201–209.

Pappas, G. and Papadimitriou, P. (2007). Challenges in *Brucella* bacteraemia. *Int. J. Antimicrob. Agents.* 30 : S29–31.

Pappas, G., Papadimitriou, P., Akritidis, N., Christou, L. and Tsianos, E.V. (2006). The new global map of human brucellosis. *Lancet Infect. Dis.* 6 : 91–99.

Paulsen, I..T., Seshadri, R., Nelson, K.E., Eisen, J.A., Heidelberg, J.F. and Read, T.D. (2002). The *Brucella suis* genome reveals fundamental similarities between animal and plant pathogens and symbionts. *Proc. Natl. Acad. Sci. USA* 99 : 13148-53.

Refai, M. (2002). Incidence and control of brucellosis in the Near East region. *Vet. Microbiol. 90* : 81-110.

Reguera, J.M., Alarcon, A., Miralles, F., Pachon, J., Juarez, C. and Colmenero, J.D. (2003). *Brucella* endocarditis: clinical, diagnostic, and therapeutic approach. *Eur. J. Clin. Microbiol. Infect. Dis.* 22 : 647–650.

Renukaradhya, G.J., Isloor, S. and Rajasekhar, M. (2002). Epidemiology, zoonotic aspects, vaccination and control/eradication of brucellosis in India. *Vet. Microbiol.* 90 : 183-95.

Robichaud, S., Libman, M., Behr, M. and Rubin, E. (2004). Prevention of laboratory-acquired brucellosis. *Clin. Infect. Dis.* 38 : e119–122.

Roth, F., Zinsstag, J., Orkhon, D., Chimed-Ochir, G., Hutton, G., Cosivi, O. (2003). Human health benefits from livestock vaccination for brucellosis: case study. *Bull W.H.O.* 81 : *867-876.*

Roushan, M.R., Gangi, S.M. and Ahmadi, S.A. (2004). Comparison of the efficacy of two months of treatment with co-trimoxazole plus doxycycline vs. co-trimoxazole plus rifampin in brucellosis. *Swiss Med. Wkly.* 134 : 564-8.

Ruiz-Mesa, J.D., Sanchez-Gonzalez, J., Reguera, J.M., Martin, L., Lopez-Palmero, S. and Colmenero, J.D. (2005). Rose Bengal test: diagnostic yield and use for the rapid diagnosis of human brucellosis in emergency departments in endemic areas. *Clin. Microbiol. Infect.* 11 : 221-5.

Sanchez, D.O., Zandomeni, R.O., Cravero, S., Verdun, R.E., Pierrou, E. and Faccio, P. (2001). Gene discovery through genomic sequencing of *Brucella abortus*. *Infect. Immun.* 69 : 865-8.

Schurig, G.G., Sriranganathan, N. and Corbel, M.J. (2002). Brucellosis vaccines: past, present and future. *Vet. Microbiol.* 90 : 479-96.

Seleem, M.N., Boyle, S.M. and Sriranganathan, N. (2008). *Brucella*: a pathogen without classic virulence genes. *Vet. Microbiol.* 129 : 1–14.

Seleem, M.N., Jain, N., Pothayee, N., Ranjan, A., Riffle, J.S. and Sriranganathan, N. (2009). Targeting *Brucella melitensis* with polymeric nanoparticles containing streptomycin and doxycycline. *FEMS Microbiol. Lett.* 294 : 24–31.

Sen, M.R., Shukla, B.N. and Goyal, R.K. (2002). Seroprevalence of brucellosis in and around Varanasi. *J. Commun. Dis.* 34 : 226-7.

Singh, S.V., Agarwal, G.S., Batra, H.V., Gupta, V.K. and Singh, N. (2000). Monitoring of *Brucella* infection associated with reproductive losses using multiple serological tests in organized goat and sheep flocks. *Indian J Anim. Sci.*70:154-6.

Smits, H.L., Abdoel, T.H., Solera, J., Clavijo, E. and Diaz, R. (2003). Immunochromatographic *Brucella*-specific immunoglobulin M and G lateral flow assays for rapid serodiagnosis of human brucellosis. *Clin. Diagn. Lab. Immunol.* 10 : 1141-6.

Solera, J. (2000). Treatment of human brucellosis. *J. Med. Liban.* 48 : 255-63.

Solera, J., Geijo, P., Largo, J., Rodriguez-Zapata, M., Gijon, J. and Martinez-Alfaro, E. (2004). A randomized, double-blind study to assess the optimal duration of doxycycline treatment for human brucellosis. *Clin. Infect. Dis.* 39 : 1776-82.

Taleski, V., Zerva, L., Kantardjiev, T. and Kirandziski, T. (2002). An overview of the epidemiology and epizootology of brucellosis in selected countries of Central and Southeast Europe. *Vet. Microbiol.* 90 :147–155.

Wattam, A.R., Williams, K.P., Snyder, E.E. and Setubal, J.C. (2009). Analysis of ten *Brucella* genomes reveals evidence for horizontal gene transfer despite a preferred intracellular lifestyle. *J. Bacteriol.* 191 : 3569–3579.

Young, E.J. (1989). *Brucellosis: clinical and laboratory aspects*. In: Corbel MJ, editor. Florida, USA: CRC Press Inc; 1989.

Young, E.J. (1995). An overview of human brucellosis. *Clin. Infect. Dis.* 21 : 283-9.

❑❑❑

14

Glanders

Synonyms : Farcy, Pacin, Carn

Glanders is a contagious, acute or chronic, usually fatal anthropo-zoonotic disease of *Equidae* caused by *Burkholderia mallei* and characterized by serial development of ulcerating nodules that are most commonly found in the upper respiratory tract, lungs, and skin. The first recorded description of glanders is from the third century from Aristotle. In 1664, glanders was recognized as a contagious disease and in 1830, it's zoonotic potential was suspected. In the late 1800's, the Mallein test (1891) was developed for diagnosis of glanders. By 1910, the U.S., Canada and Great Britain all implemented glanders-control programs. *B. mallei* was eradicated from the United States in 1929.

Etiology : It is caused by *Burkholderia mallei*. It is a straight or slightly bent Gm – non-spore forming, non-motile rod. The organisms in old culture appear as pleomorphic. The organisms can grow in ordinary media but addition of defrinated horse blood or glycerol accelerate the growth. Colonies have hop like odour and slime consistency. The organisms are readily destroyed by direct sunlight and most of the disinfectants. They can survive for 20 days in water and 6 weeks in contaminated stable. This organism is closely related to the agent of melioidosis, *Burkholderia pseudomallei*.

Susceptible hosts: The most susceptible hosts are horses, mules and donkeys. Infections can also occur in dogs, cats, goats and camels; cats may be particularly susceptible. Hamsters and guinea pigs can be infected in the laboratory. It is an occupational / professional hazard to human being. Laboratory samples are highly infectious to humans. Infection have been observed in sheep and goats. Guinea pigs, rabbits and field mice may be infected fatally. Cattle and pigs are absolutely resistant.

Geographic Distribution : Glanders is seen in some Middle Eastern countries, the Indian subcontinent, Southeast Asia, parts of China and Mongolia, and Africa. Sporadic cases are also seen in South America.

Sporadic cases of glanders were identified between 1985-86 to 1990-91 from the states of Haryana, Himachal Pradesh and Punjab. Since reemergence of glanders in July – August 2006 in and around Pune and Panchgani area of Maharastra, several cases have been reported among equines of different states viz., Andhra Pradesh, Uttar Pradesh, Uttarakhand, Punjab. During the year 2006-07, National Research Centre on Equines, Hissar tested 4395 samples and 97 were detected positive and *B. mallei* was isolated from 8 of these cases.

Transmission : Transmission is usually by ingestion in horses and related species; the infection can also be spread by inhalation or through skin abrasions and the conjunctiva. Carnivores can become infected after eating contaminated meat. *B. mallei* is spread on fomites, including harnesses, grooming tools, food and water troughs. Outside the host, the organism has little resistance to drying, heat, light or chemicals, so that survival beyond 2 weeks is unlikely. Under favourable conditions, however, it can probably survive a few months. *Burkholderia mallei* can remain viable in tap water for at least 1 month. For disinfection, benzalkonium chloride or 'roccal' (1/2000), sodium hypochlorite (500 ppm available chlorine), iodine, mercuric chloride in alcohol, and potassium permanganate have been shown to be highly effective against *B. mallei*. Phenolic disinfectants are less effective.

Humans can become infected after contact with sick animals or infectious materials. Transmission is typically through small wounds and abrasions in the skin; ingestion or inhalation, with invasion through the mucous membranes, is also possible. Cases are usually seen in people who handle laboratory samples or have frequent close contact with horses, mules and donkeys. Natural human infections are rare even when infection rates in horses are 5–30%. Humans are not highly susceptible and infection may gain access through skin abrasions to produce granulomatous disease and pyemia. The case fatality rate is high. *B. mallei* has been attempted by some countries as biological weapon.

Pathogenesis : In animal, after natural infections, the incubation period varies from 6 days to many months; 2 to 6 weeks is typical. Experimental infections can result in clinical signs after 3 days. In human, after natural infections, the incubation period is 1 to14 days. Infections from aerosolized forms in biological weapons are expected to have an incubation period of 10–14 days. On gaining access through intestinal mucosa the organisms set up septicaemia in acute form and bacterimia in chronic form. They may invade the regional lymph nodes. On entrance through skin, organisms would reach blood stream, localize in various organs and forms nodes and ulcers in skin. Involvement of lungs leads to typical signs of broncho-pneumonia.

Clinical Signs: a. In animal:

Acute, chronic and latent forms of glanders are seen in horses, mules and donkeys. Donkeys are more susceptible to *B. mallei* and are therefore more likely to develop the acute form of disease. Horses are more resistant than donkeys, and tend to develop the chronic form of the disease. Mules are intermediate in susceptibility. Immunocompromised or undernourished animals and those kept in unsanitary conditions are at higher risk of developing disease.

In acute form, animals usually have septicemia and high fever (up to 106°F / 41°C) and, subsequently, a thick, mucopurulent nasal discharge and respiratory signs. Death occurs within a few days. The chronic disease is common in horses and is seen as a debilitating condition with nodular or ulcerative cutaneous and nasal lesions. Infected animals may live for years and disseminate the organism. The prognosis is unfavorable. Recovered animals may not develop immunity. In the latent form, there may be few symptoms other than a nasal discharge and occasional labored breathing. Lesions may be found only in the lungs.

Nasal, pulmonary, and cutaneous forms of glanders are recognized, and an animal may be affected by more than one form at a time. In the nasal form, nodules develop in the mucosa of the nasal septum and lower parts of the turbinates. The nodules degenerate into deep ulcers with raised irregular borders. Characteristic star-shaped cicatrices remain after the ulcers heal. In the early stage, the submaxillary lymph nodes are enlarged and edematous, and later become adherent to the skin or deeper tissues.

In the pulmonary form, small tubercle-like nodules, which have caseous or calcified centers surrounded by inflammatory zones, are found in the lungs. If the disease process is extensive, consolidation of the lung tissue and pneumonia may be present. The nodules tend to break down and may discharge their contents into the bronchioles, resulting in extension of the infection to the upper respiratory tract.

In the cutaneous form ("farcy"), nodules appear along the course of the lymph vessels, particularly of the extremities. These nodules degenerate and form ulcers that discharge a highly infectious, sticky pus. Lymphatic vessels may become filled and distended with pus, and may be referred to as "Farcy pipes". The liver and spleen also may show typical nodular lesions.

b. In human:

Humans can develop four forms of disease: septicemia, pulmonary infection and acute localized infection or chronic infection. Combinations of syndromes can also occur. In the septicemic form, fever, chills, myalgia, and pleuritic chest pain develop acutely. Other symptoms may include generalized erythroderma, jaundice, photophobia, lacrimation, diarrhea and granulomatous or necrotizing lesions. Tachycardia, cervical adenopathy and mild hepatomegaly or splenomegaly may also be seen. Death usually occurs in 7 to 10 days.

The pulmonary form is characterized by symptoms of pneumonia, pulmonary abscesses and pleural infusions. A cough, fever, dyspnea and mucopurulent discharge may be seen. Skin abscesses sometimes develop after several months.

Localized infections are characterized by nodules, abscesses and ulcers in the mucous membranes, skin, lymphatic vessels and/or subcutaneous tissues. A mucopurulent, blood–tinged discharge may be seen from the mucous membranes. The lymph nodes may be swollen. Mucosal or skin infections can disseminate; symptoms of disseminated infections include a papular or pustular rash, abscesses in the internal organs (particularly the liver and spleen) and pulmonary lesions. Disseminated infections are associated with septic shock and high mortality. In the chronic form, multiple abscesses, nodules or ulcers can be seen in the skin, liver, spleen or muscles.

The septicemic form has a high mortality rate in humans: the case fatality rate is 95% in untreated cases and more than 50% when the infection is treated. The mortality rate for localized disease is 20% when treated. The overall mortality rate is 40%.

Lesions : At necropsy, there may be ulcers, nodules and stellate scars in the nasal cavity, trachea, pharynx, larynx, skin and subcutaneous tissues. Catarrhal bronchopneumonia with enlarged bronchial lymph nodes may be evident. The lungs, liver, spleen and kidneys may contain firm, rounded, and encapsulated miliary gray nodules similar to tubercles. The lymphatic vessels may be swollen; the lymph nodes are typically enlarged and fibrotic and contain focal abscesses. In addition, necrosis may be noted in the internal organs and testes. *B. mallei* and sometimes along with *Arcanobacterium pyogens* are isolated from the infected tissue.

Diagnosis : It is based on the clinical signs and pathological lesions. However, for confirmatory diagnosis following tests are carried out.

1. Identification of the agent

The glanders should be differentiated on the basis of clinical symptoms from other chronic infections of the nasal mucosae or sinuses, and from strangles (*Streptococcus equi*), ulcerative lymphangitis (*Corynebacterium pseudotuberculosis*), pseudotuberculosis (*Yersinia pseudotuberculosis*) and sporotrichosis (*Sporotrichium* spp.). Glanders should be excluded positively from suspected cases of epizootic lymphangitis (*Histoplasma farciminosum*), with which it has many clinical similarities. In humans in particular, glanders should be distinguished from melioidosis (*B. pseudomallei*).

a. Morphology of *B. mallei*

The smears from fresh lesions on methylene blue or Gram staining show numerous organisms, but in older lesions they are scanty. The organisms are mainly extracellular, fairly straight Gram-negative rods with rounded ends, 2-5 μm long and 0.3-0.8 μm wide with no flagellae. The presence of a capsule-like cover, composed of neutral carbohydrates, has been established by electron microscopy. The organisms, in tissue sections, have a beaded appearance.

b. Cultural characteristics

The organism is aerobic and facultatively anaerobic only in the presence of nitrate, growing optimally at 37°C. It grows well, but slowly (48-hour incubation), on ordinary culture media; glycerol enrichment is particularly useful. After a few days on glycerol agar, there is a confluent, slightly cream-coloured growth that is smooth, moist, and viscid. With continued incubation, the growth thickens and becomes dark brown and tough. It also grows well on glycerol potato agar and in glycerol broth, on which a slimy pellicle forms. On plain nutrient agar, the growth is much less luxuriant, and growth is poor on gelatin. In culture media, they vary in appearance depending on the age of the culture and type of medium. In older cultures, it is pleomorphic and branching filaments form on the surface of broth cultures.

Alterations to characteristics may occur *in vitro*, so fresh isolates should be used for identification reactions. Litmus milk is slightly acidified by *B. mallei*, and coagulation may occur after long incubation. Glucose and other carbohydrates, such as arabinose, fructose, galactose and mannose, are consistently fermented by *B. mallei*. Indole is not produced, horse blood is not haemolysed and no diffusible pigments are produced in cultures.

In contaminated samples, supplementation of media with substances that inhibit the growth of Gram-positive organisms (e.g. crystal violet, proflavine) has proved useful, as has pretreatment with penicillin (1000 units/ml for 3 hours at 37°C). A selective medium composed of polymyxin E (1000 units), bacitracin (250 units), and actidione (0.25 mg) incorporated into nutrient agar (100 ml) containing glycerine (4%), donkey or horse serum (10%), and ovine haemoglobin or trypton agar (0.1%) can be used.

c. Laboratory animal inoculation

Guinea-pigs, hamsters and cats have been used for diagnosis. For isolation of the organism suspected material is inoculated intraperitoneally into a male guinea-pig. Positive material will give rise to a severe localised peritonitis and orchitis (Strauss reaction). The Strauss reaction is not specific for glanders and other organisms can elicit it.

d. Molecular biological techniques

There have been recent advances in the application of molecular biological techniques to the detection of glanders. Conventional polymerase chain reaction (PCR), real-time PCR, PCR-RFLP for the specific detection of *B. mallei* DNA has been developed that allows differentiation between *B. mallei* and *B. pseudomallei*. The technique has not yet been fully validated or gained wide acceptance. However, PCR has the potential to be a safe, fast method to confirm infection.

2. Mallein tests

The mallein purified protein derivative (PPD) is a solution of water-soluble protein fractions of heat-treated *B. mallei*. The test depends on infected horses being hypersensitive to mallein. Advanced clinical cases in horses and acute cases in donkeys and mules may give inconclusive results requiring additional methods of diagnosis to be employed.

a. The intradermo-palpebral test

This is the most sensitive, reliable and specific test for detecting infected equidae, and has largely displaced the ophthalmic and subcutaneous tests: 0.1 ml of concentrated mallein PPD is injected intradermally into the lower eyelid and the test is read at 24 and 48 hours. A positive reaction is characterized by marked oedematous swelling of the eyelid, and there may be a purulent discharge from the inner canthus or conjunctiva. This is usually accompanied by a rise in temperature. With a negative response, there is usually no reaction or only a little swelling of the lower lid.

b. The ophthalmic test

A few drops of mallein are instilled into the eye at the canthus. In an infected animal, the eyelids, and sometimes the side of the face, become swollen and there may be a little discharge from the eye. The reaction may also occur to a lesser extent in the opposite eye.

c. The subcutaneous test

This test interferes with subsequent serological diagnosis, and not be acceptable in some countries also. The horse's temperature has to be under 102°F (38.8°C) on the day before the test, at the time of the injection, and at 9, 12 and 15 hours after the injection. A 10 cm square skin patch in the middle of the neck is clipped and disinfected; 2.5 ml of dilute mallein are injected subcutaneously into the centre of the patch. With a positive test, the horse develops a pyrexia of 104°F (40.0°C) or over during the first 15 hours, and a firm painful swelling with raised edges develops within 24 hours at the injection site. In nonglandered horses, there is no, or minimal, transient local swelling. Doubtful reactors may be retested after 14 days using a double dose of mallein.

3. Serological tests

a. Complement fixation test

CF test is not as sensitive as the mallein test but is an accurate serological test that has been used for glanders diagnosis for many years and is a prescribed test for international trade. It is reported to be 90-95% accurate, serum being positive within 1 week of infection and remaining positive in the case of exacerbation of the chronic process. The antigen used is primarily lipopolysaccharide. The young culture of *B. mallei* heated for 1 hour at 70°C can be used as antigen, which must be tested for safety by inoculating on blood agar plates before use.

A sample that produces 100% haemolysis at the 1/5 dilution is negative, 25-75% haemolysis is suspicious, and no haemolysis (100% fixation) is positive. Unfortunately, false-positive results can occur due to cross reaction between *B. pseudomallei* and *B. mallei*. Also healthy horses can have a false positive CF reaction for a variable period following a mallein intradermal test.

b. Enzyme-linked immunosorbent assays

Both plate and membrane (blot) enzyme-linked immunosorbent assays (ELISAs) have been reported for the serodiagnosis of glanders, but none of these procedures has been shown to differentiate serologically between *B. mallei* and *B. pseudomallei*. Blotting approaches have involved both dipstick dot-blot and electrophoretically separated and transferred western blot methods. A competitive ELISA that uses an anti-lipopolysaccharide monoclonal antibody has also been developed and found to be similar to the CF test in performance. The development of monoclonal antibody reagents specific for *B. mallei* antigenic components offers the potential for more specific ELISAs in the foreseeable future that will help resolve questionable test results of quarantined imported horses.

The avidin-biotin dot ELISA has been described, but has not yet been widely used or validated. The antigen is heat-inactivated bacterial culture that has been concentrated and purified. A dot of this antigen is placed on a nitrocellulose dipstick that is then used to test for antibody against *B. mallei* in equine serum. Using antigen-dotted, preblocked dipsticks, the test can be completed in approximately 1 hour. Serum or whole blood can be used for the test, and partial haemolysis does not impart any background colour to the antigen-coated area on the nitrocellulose.

Recombinant protein antigen based ELISA for serodiagnosis of glandes is also under the stage of development and validity.

c. Other serological tests

The rose bengal plate agglutination test (RBT) has been described for the diagnosis of glanders in horses and other susceptible animals; the test has been validated in Russia only. The antigen is a heat-inactivated bacterial suspension coloured with rose bengal, which is used in a plate agglutination test. The accuracy of other agglutination tests and precipitin is unsatisfactory for use in control programmes. Horses with chronic glanders and those in a debilitated condition give negative or inconclusive results.

Treatment and Vaccination

Glanders is a notifiable disease under Glanders and Farcy act. As per the act, the animals declared positive must be destroyed and safely disposed. Penicillin and streptomycin have no effect. But Na sulfadiazine for 20 days has been highly effective in the treatment of experimental glanders causing 100% recovery. Combination of a formalized preparation of *B. mallei* and sulfadiazine or mallein and sulfadimidine are reported to be effective in the treatment of affected horses. However, treatment is not generally recommended, as infections can be spread to humans and other animals, and treated animals may become asymptomatic carriers. Vaccines are not available.

Control

Animals with clinical evidence of glanders and those positive to mallein test or CFT must be regarded as diseased and should be destroyed and disposed off cautiously as follows:

a. The carcasses must be deep buried or better incinerated.

b. The premises should be vigorously disinfected.

c. All the in contacts, suspected and imported animals must be isolated, properly tested and all positive reactors must be destroyed and their carcasses incinerated.

d. Manure, beddings, feed residue should be burnt and buried.

e. The research works on *B. mallei* must be carried out under bio-safety level 3 containment precautions.

Further reading

Al-Ani, F. K. and Al-Delaimi, A. K. (1988). Epizootic lymphangitis in horses: clinical, epidemiological and hematological studies. *Pakistan Vet. J.* 6: 96-100.

Al-Ani, F. K., Al-Delami, A. K. and Ali A. H. (1987) Glanders in horses: clinical and epidemiological studies in Iraq. *Pakistan Vet. J.* 79: 126-129.

Al-Ani, F. K, Ali, A. and Banna, H. H. B. (1992): Glanders in horses: histopathological and electron microscopic studies. *Pakistan Vet. J.* 12: 1-3.

Al-Ani, F. K., Al-Omran, A. H. and Al-Zubaidy, F. S. (1993). A micro-enzyme-linked immunosorbent assay (ELISA) for detection of antibody to *Pseudomonas mallei* infection in horses. *Pakistan Vet. J.* 13: 70-73.

Al-Ani, F. K., O. F. Al-Rawsashdeh, H. A. and Ali, F. K. Hassan. (1998): Glanders in horses: clinical, biochemical and serological studies in Iraq. *Vet. Arhiv.* 68 : 155-162.

Al-Kafawi, A. A., Al-Ani, F. K., Al-Bassam, L. S. and Youkob, A. Y. (1977). Hematological changes in Arabian horses infected with glanders. *Vet. Rec.* 101: 427.

Alibasoglu, M., T. Yesildere, T., Calislar, Inal, T. and Calsikan, U. (1986): Glanders outbreak in lions in the Istanbul zoological garden. *Berl. Münch. Tierärtzl. Wschr.* 99: 57-63.

Ballarini, G. (1985). Glanders: a danger still present. *Obiettivi Documenti Vet.* 6: 41-43.

Batmanov, V. P., Iliukhin, V. I., Lozovaia, N. A. and Iakovlev, A. T. (1996): Recovery rate in chemotherapy of glanders. *Antibiot. Khimioter.* 41: 30-34.

Blancou, J. (1994a): Early methods for the surveillance and control of glanders in *Europe. Rev. Sci. Tech.* 13: 545-557.

Blancou, J. (1994b): Historical methods for the monitoring and control of glanders. *Bull.*

Mensuel dela Soc. Vet. Prat. France. 78: 45-54.

Dance, D. A.(2000): Melioidosis as an emerging global problem. *Acta. Trop.* 74: 115-119.

Al-Ani, K. F and Roberson, J. (2007). Glanders in horses: A review of the literature. *Vet. Arhiv.* 77 (3): 203-218.

Fathi, R., Barafroukut, A. Charaf, Y. and Fekraf, M. (1953). Treatment of glanders in horses by sulfamethazine. *Arch. Instit. Hessarek.* **7:** 22-26.

Gee, J. E., Sacchi, C. T., Glass, M. B., De, B. K., Weyant, R. S., Levett, P. N. and Whitney, A. M. (2003). Use of 16S rRNA gene sequencing for rapid identification and differentiation of *Burkholderia pseudomallei* and *B. mallei. J. Clin. Microbiol.* 41: 4647-4654.

Godoy, D., Randle, G., Simpson, A. J. Aanensen, D. M., Pitt, T. L., Kinoshita, R. and Spratt, B. G. (2003). Multilocus sequence typing and evolutionary relationships among the causative agents of melioidosis and glanders, *Burkholderia pseudomallei* and *Burkholderia mallei*. *J. Clin. Microbiol.* 41: 2068-2079.

Hagebock, J. M., Schlater, L. K., Frerichs, W. M. and Olson, D P. (1993): Serologic responses to the mallein test for glanders in solipeds. *J. Vet. Diag. Invest.* 5: 97-99.

❑❑❑

15

Hemorrhagic Septicaemia

Synonyms : Pasteurellosis, shipping fever, Stockyardis disease, Stockyardis pneumonia, Barbone disease

Hemorrhagic septicaemia is a particular form of pasteurellosis caused by *Pasteurella multocida* and manifested by an acute and highly fatal septicaemia mainly in cattle and water buffaloes. The disease includes pneumonic pasteurellosis (shipping or transport fever), a disease caused mainly by *P. haemolytica*, although various serotypes of *P. multocida* are occasionally involved. Although the morbidity of pneumonic pasteurellosis of cattle can be high, the mortality rate is much less than that of hemorrhagic septicemia. Hemorrhagic septicaemia is caused by two serotypes of *P. multocida* namely, B:2 and E:2. The letter denotes the capsular antigen as determined originally by the indirect hemagglutination test of Carter, and the numeral 2 stands for the somatic or O antigen as determined by the agar gel diffusion-precipitin test developed by Heddelston and associates. This somatic antigen 2 is the equivalent to the 6 in the classification of Namioka and associates. In a new classification, *Pasteurella multocida* strains causing most pasteurella infections, including hemorrhagic septicemia, are called *P. multocida* subspecies *multocida*. Haemorrhagic septicaemia (HS) has a wide distribution particularly in tropical countries in Africa and Asia. In Asia, HS epidemics may occur as an alarming and devastating disease problems in cattle and buffaloes causing enormous economic losses.

Within the Asian Region, countries can be classified into three categories, on the basis of incidence and distribution of the disease : endemic or sporadic, clinically sus-pected but not confirmed, or free. Most Asian countries rank HS as the most important contagious disease or the most important bacterial disease in cattle and buffaloes.

Etiology : It is a Gram negative coccoid, short rod or filamentous shaped organism and takes a bipolar staining following Leishman or Methylene blue stain. The organism is a normal inhabitant of upper respiratory tract and may not be able to produce disease alone. But predisposing factors like fatigue, transportation, over exertion, starvation, close confinement to damp and humid atmosphere may help the organism to assume virulent role and set up the disease process. The organism produces an endotoxin. The organism is easily killed by usual disinfectants.

Geographical distribution : The disease is reported to be endemic and is of utmost economic importance in Bhutan, China, India, Indonesia, Mongolia, Myanmar, Philippines, Sri Lanka and Malaysia. Most of these countries have large cattle/buffalo populations. Furthermore, livestock rearing is largely extensive and management is rather poor in view of the significance of ruminants in the respective national economies. Sporadic outbreaks of the disease have been suspected clinically in Kuwait, Qatar but not confirmed by isolation of the agent and serotyping. These countries are net livestock importers and the disease is introduced occasionally through cattle imports. Presently, Singapore, Chinese Province of Hong Kong, Israel are free of the disease and the disease has never been reported in Japan and Jordan.

Pathogenesis : The incubation period is 2-5 days. The pasteurella organisms remain as commensal in the terminal bronchiole and alveoli. The organisms assume the virulent role due to stress imposed by predisposing factors like transportation, malnutrition and climatic changes.

Transmission : The disease is spread by direct and indirect contact (fomites). The source of the infection is infected animals or carriers. The carrier state may be greater than 20 percent shortly after an outbreak, but within 6 weeks the rate is usually less than 5 percent. The causal agent does not survive for more than 2 to 3 weeks in the soil or on pastures. Close herding and wetness, as occurs during the rainy season appear to contribute to spread.

Incubation Period : The influence of extrinsic factors in the development of the clinical pasteurellosis, and particularly in hemorrhagic septicemia, has been noted by many workers. When favourable circumstances for the growth and multiplication of *P. multocida* in the animal body occur, severe septicemia develops within a few hours. However, the organisms may be harboured for varying periods in a small percentage of carrier animals without any clinical sign. The perpetuation of the disease from year to year or season to season is generally attributed to the carrier state. The immune status of the animal is thought to influence the severity of the disease. Cattle or buffalo artificially inoculated subcutaneously with lethal doses (approximately 20,000 bacilli) show clinical signs within a few hours and succumb within 18 to 30 hours.

Clinical signs : The majority of cases in cattle and buffaloes are acute or peracute with death occurring from 6 to 24 hours after the first recognized signs. In a few outbreaks, animals may survive as long as 72 hours. Dullness, reluctance to move and elevated temperature are the first signs. Following these signs, salivation and nasal discharge appear, and edematous swellings are seen in the pharyngeal region and then spread to the ventral cervical region and brisket. Visible mucous membranes are congested, and respiratory distress is soon followed by collapse and death. Recovery, particularly in buffaloes, is rare. Chronic manifestations of hemorrhagic septicaemia do not appear to occur.

Gross Lesions : Widely distributed hemorrhages, edema, and general hyperemia are the most obvious tissue changes observed in infected animals. In almost all cases there is an edematous swelling of the head, neck, and brisket region. Incision of the edematous swellings reveals a coagulated serofibrinous mass with straw colored or blood-stained fluid. This edema, which distends tissue spaces, is also found in the musculature. There are subserosal petechial haemorrhages throughout the animal, and blood-tinged fluid is frequently found in the thoracic and abdominal cavities. Petechiae may be found scattered throughout some tissues and lymph nodes, particularly the pharyngeal and cervical nodes, which are also swollen and often hemorrhagic. Pneumonia is not usually extensive and gastroenteritis is usually absent or mild. Cases that are atypical in regard to throat swelling (absent) and pneumonia (extensive) are occasionally seen.

Epidemiology : H.S. is considered an economically important disease in Southern Europe, Russia, Africa, Near East, Middle East, South Africa, India and South and South East Asia including Indonesia, Malayasia, Thailand, Philippines causing huge economic losses. The major susceptible animal species consist of cattle and buffaloes. Buffaloes are more susceptible than cattle and that, in both species, young and young adult animals are more susceptible than older animals. Animals of all ages are susceptible but animals of 6 months to 2 years are most susceptible. The case fatality rates vary from 50-100% and depends on the immune status of the herd. The case fatality rate for buffaloes is 3 times more compared to cattle. The disease usually occurs in wet humid weather during rainy season. During intervening period the causative organisms persist on the tonsillar and nasopharyngeal mucosae of carrier animals. Approximately 45% of healthy cattle in herds are associated with the disease whereas 3-5% of cattle from herds are unassociated with the disease. Spread occurs through inhalation of organisms from clinically normal carriers or clinical cases or ingestion of contaminated food stuff. The saliva of affected animals contains large numbers of Pasteurella organisms and it remains viable for more than 24 h in the pasture. The two common serotypes of *Pasteurella multocida* associated with disease in these species are types B:2 (in Asia) and E:2 (in Africa). The Asian B:2 serotype has also been associated with sporadic septicaemic disease in pigs. Besides type B:2, several other B serotypes have been incriminated in sporadic outbreaks of disease particularly in feral ruminants. The organism causing HS does not survive outside the animal body to any significant degree so as to be a source of infection. Moist conditions prolong its survival. Thus the disease tends to spread more during the wet season. The onset of the monsoon in Asian countries also set into motion other activities such as rice cultivation which bring about movements of animals, work stress in work animals, etc. all of which favour the precipitation of outbreaks. Infection occurs by inhalation or ingestion of *P. multocida* bacteria. Higher incidence of HS is associated with moist, humid conditions, high buffalo population density, and extensive free grazing system of management, where large herds graze freely in common pastures and are kept together at night. In situations where occasional sporadic outbreaks occur in some regions within endemic countries, mortality may be very high unlike endemic areas where regular, seasonal outbreaks occur, where losses in each outbreak are low and confined to young animals. The phenomenon of naturally acquired immunity resulting from the so-called non-fatal infection largely controls the mortality and morbidity patterns. The animals that have recovered from HS acquire a long lasting carrier status which render the prevention of new outbreaks rather difficult. These losses in endemic areas may be of an insidious nature which may escape the notice of the animal health authorities but may be of considerable economic significance. Once clinical signs appear, case fatality is nearly 100%. Variable numbers of immune carriers are present in animal populations, particularly in endemic areas. They may be latent carriers, where the organisms are lodged in the tonsils, or active carriers, where organisms are detectable in the nasopharynx.

Diagnosis : The clinical, provisional diagnosis of HS is based on a combination of clinical signs, gross pathological lesions and a consideration of relevant epidemiological parameters and other similar diseases prevalent in the locality. A provisional diagnosis is important since preventive measures to control the spread of the disease are required immediately, without waiting for the necessary laboratory confirmation. At the earliest opportunity, however, appropriate material should be collected and dispatched to the nearest laboratory. The mere isolation of *P. multocida* does not mean that HS is diagnosed. On the one hand it should be put in the epidemiological context and, on the other hand the isolated strain must be serotyped. Anthrax, black quarter should always be considered when investigating sudden deaths in cattle and buffaloes. A variety of diagnostic techniques have been developed over the years for HS. These include:

(a) Blood smear, culture and biological tests for isolation of the causative agent. Mouse isolation may prove necessary as samples are often heavily contaminated when they reach the diagnostic laboratory. A mouse colony is therefore necessary in such laboratories.

(b) Biochemical and serological tests (capsular such as rapid slide agglutination and indirect haemagglutination tests or somatic such as agar gel pre-cipitation test) for identification of *P. multocida* and determination of serotypes. An ELISA test has recently been developed in Australia, however it fails to differentiate between the Asian (B:2) and African (E:2) types. This is not a serious limitation in Asia as only B:2 type of *P. multocida* has been encountered so far. Thus ELISA can be a good test for screening a large number of cultures from a collection in a laboratory where the turnover is high.

(c) Nonserological tests for presumptive identification of serotypes (e.g. acriflavine flocculation test, hyaluronidase test).

(d) Molecular methods such as PCR, ribotyping or restriction endonuclease analysis which have an epidemiological significance because they enable strain differentiation within serotypes and hence some epidemiological inferences, for investigations extending beyond routine diagnosis.

Treatment : The HS is a primary bacterial disease and, theoretically, could be effectively treated by the wide range of antibiotics currently available. However, treatment is constrained by a host of practical considerations. Animals can be cured only if they have been treated in the very early stages of the disease. The conditions for an early detection of the disease and hence its effective treatment are usually lacking in primitive husbandry systems. In organised farms, however, early detection and effective treatment are achieved through regular checking of rectal temperatures of in-contact animals. Either streptomycin or oxytetracycline may be administered by intramuscular route at fairly high dosage. Penicillin and Ampicillin are also widely used. Antibiotic resistance of *P. multocida* may occur and it has been reported at least vis-à-vis streptomycin and sulphonamides.

Prevention and control : Vaccination is a major control measure in the face of a new epidemic. Various vaccine types have been developed : which the broth bacterin, the oil adjuvant vaccine, the double emulsion vaccine and a live vaccine. The latter is a deer strain aerosol vaccine developed in Myanmar. Although this vaccine is the sole vaccine used (apparently with success) in Myanmar, it does not seem to have gained popular acceptance outside this country. The reasons advanced to explain this are numerous: the fact that the strain concerned (*Pasteurella multocida* serotype B:3.4) has occasionally been associated with sporadic outbreaks of disease and its occasional virulence to young animals when administered by the subcutaneous route are the possible reasons, apart from the general reluctance to use a live vaccine and the fact that antibiotics cannot be administered simultaneously to this live vaccine. During an outbreak, one should resort to immediate whole herd vaccination, irrespective of previous vaccination history. The use of either broth bacterin or oil adjuvant vaccine is recom-mended. Sanitary measures include early detection and isolation of new cases and their immediate treatment with antibiotics, deep burial of carcasses or incineration, and the prevention of movements of animals to disease free areas.

In endemic areas vaccination should be carried out on a routine prophylactic basis preferably two to three months before the high-risk season (monsoon). Awareness of the disease among farmers backed up by a good disease reporting/disease information system should be adopted. The animals from endemic and nonendemic areas should be segregated to avoid contact with carriers.

While importing the animals, following guidelines should be followed. Briefly, these are : (a) ensure that the animals originate from a region where no outbreaks of HS have occurred for a minimum period of one year; (b) carry out an indirect haemagglutination (IHA) testing (a test which can reveal recent infection) on the animals to be exported as well as on a random sample of in-contacts in the country of origin whenever possible (c) hold animals under observation for 2–3 weeks before transport (while carrying out the above testing) (d) quarantine them for the same period of time upon arrival to destination and (e) vaccinate all animals at the end of the quarantine period. Whenever animals are exported from HS endemic countries, even after observing all the above precautions, it is important to vaccinate all susceptible stock in the importing country that are likely to come into contact with the imported animals.

Economy of the disease : HS is a disease of utmost economic importance particularly in Asia and to a lesser extent in Africa. In Asia the susceptible animal population consists of 432 million cattle and 146 million buffaloes, which constitute 30% and 95% of the world's cattle and buffalo population, respectively. In India where the production of milk is highest in Asia, around 50% of the milk come from the more susceptible buffaloes. In Asia as a whole, the contribution of the buffalo to the milk production is 37%. Most of the cattle and buffaloes are used as draught animals in the rice fields, and rice is the staple diet in many countries. Thus, the high population of buffaloes in Asia, the high susceptibility of buffalo to HS and the high case fatality, all point to the significance of the economic losses due to the disease. Few countries have attempted to quantify the losses due to HS, and there is no uniformity in the methods adopted. Thus, these studies are not strictly comparable, but will reflect the trends. Most of the available information is derived from passive reporting systems. In India, annual economic loss due to HS is around Rs. 225 million. During the past four decades it has been found that HS accounted for 46–55% of all bovine deaths. During the twelve years period since 1974 to 1986 it accounted for 58.7% of the aggregate of deaths due to five endemic diseases, viz. foot-and-mouth disease (FMD), rinderpest, blackquarter, anthrax and HS. In an active surveillance study in Sri Lanka, it was shown that in the 1970's, around 15% buffaloes and 8% cattle in the HS endemic areas died of HS annually. During the same period, the passive reporting systems recorded only 1 200 to 1 500 deaths a year in a cattle and buffalo population of approximately 2.5 million. Other countries in South Asia also ranked HS as the most economically important infectious disease or the most economically important bacterial disease. Pakistan reports that 34.4% of all deaths in susceptible stock are due to HS. With a cattle and buffalo population of 17.7 and 18.8 million respectively, the annual economic losses have been estimated at 1.89 billion rupees (350 million USD).

In the South-East Asian region, countries such as Indonesia, Malaysia, Thailand, Myanmar, Laos, Cambodia and the Philippines rank HS high among the economically important diseases of cattle and buffaloes. In Myanmar it is reckoned that 50% of the government's effort in animal disease control is directed towards HS. Malaysia, with a relatively small population of 735 000 cattle and 186 000 buffaloes, estimates the animal losses due to HS to be 0.85 million USD. Most estimates of losses take into account only direct losses, i.e. value of animals that die of HS. A true estimate of losses should take into account a variety of factors which constitute indirect losses. These are listed below:

(i) Loss of productivity – milk, meat, draught power, and cost of alternate sources of draught power.

(ii) Impairment of the reproductive potential of the animals.

(iii) A reliable differential diagnosis as there is tendency during the monsoon to attribute any mortality to HS. Thus a possible over-estimation of these losses should be taken into account. However, it must also be borne in mind that reported losses constitute only a fraction of the actual losses. This is bound to be so since HS is a disease that occurs in situations where husbandry practices are poor and therefore disease reporting system will also be poorly developed.

Measures to check the disease : Simple, accurate and rapid diagnostic tests should be developed that can be carried out even in the modestly equipped laboratories in the region. Techniques should be standardised. A Manual of Diagnostic Procedures should be prepared. Sufficient knowledge of the epidemiology of the disease should be acquired in particular country so as to formulate a strategic control programme. Disease reporting and surveillance systems in general should be strengthened. Protocols for collection of relevant epidemiological data should be developed and the management and processing of such data so as to obtain a clear epidemiological picture in each country. Development of a strategic vaccination programme for each country based on the above information should be assisted. Training programmes for veterinarians and other animal health field officers must be carried out at a regular basis to contain the spread of the disease. Also, awareness among the livestock farmers must be enhanced so as to improve their co-operation and their participation encouraged in the control programme. This would require a serious investment towards the improvement of the quality of the veterinary extension services.

Further reading

Animal Health Information Services (1997). Deputy Commissioner (LH). Department of Animal Health, Ministry of Agriculture, Govt. of India, New Delhi, India.

Aye, P.P., Angrick, T.Y., Morishita and Harr, B.S. (2001). Prevalence and characteristics of *Pasteurella multocida* : a review. *Avian Dis.* 45(1) : 182-190.

Blackall, P.J. and Miflin, J.K. (2000). Identification and typing of *Pasterurella multocida* : a review. *Avian Pathol.* 29 : 271-287.

Dabo, S.M., Confer, A.W. and Quijano, B. (2003). Molecular and immunological characterization of *Pasteurella multocida* serotype A:3 OmpA : evidence of its role in *P. multocida* interaction with extracellular matrix molecules. *Microb. Pathog.* 35: 147-157.

De Alwis, M.C. L. (1996). Haemorrhagic septicaemia : clinical and epidemiological features of the disease Proc. International Workshop on Diagnosis and Control of HS, Bali, Indonesia, May 28-30.

De Alwis, M.C.L., Arawwawela, C.B. and Vipulasiri, A.A. (1981). Formulation of a suitable medium for obtaining dense cultures for haemorrhagic septicaemia vaccine production. *Ceylon Vet. J.* 29(1-4) : 16-19.

De Alwis, M.C.L., Wijewardana, T.G., Gomis, A.I.U. and Vipulasiri, A.A. (1990). Persistence of the carrier state in haemorrhagic septicaemia *(Pasteurella multocida). Vet. Med. Czech.* 47: 234–240.

De Alwis, Wijewardana, T.G., Gomis, A.I.U. and Vipulasiri, A.A. (1990). Persistence of a carrier status in haemorrhagic septicaemia (*Pasteurella multocida* serotype 6:B) in buffaloes. *Trop. Anim. Hlth Prod.* 22 : 185-194.

Dutta, J., Rathore, B.S., Mullik, S.G., Singh, R. and Sharma, G.C. (1990). Epidemiological studies and occurrence of haemorrhagic septicaemia in India. *Indian Vet. J.* 67: 893–899.

Dutta, T.K., Gautam, R., Kumar, V.S. S. and Kotwal, S.K. (2005)., *J. Res. (SKUAST).* 4 : 13-24.

Joseph, S., Thomas, N., Singh, S, Thangapandian, E., Kumar, A.A., Singh, V.P. and Srivastava, S.K. (2007). Genetic polymorphism in the type 4 fimbrial gene (ptfA) of *Pasteurella multocida* serogroups. *Indian Vet. J.* 84: 794-797.

Kamp, E.M., Bokken, G.C., Vermeulen, T.M., deJong, M.F., Buys, H.E., Reek, F.H. and Smith, M.A. (1996). A specific and sensitive PCR assay suitable for large scale detection of toxigenic *Pasteurella multocida* nasal and tonsillar swab specimens of pigs. *J. Vet. Diag. Invest.* 8 : 304-309.

Kedrak, A. and Borkowska-Opacka B. (2001). Phenotypic characteristics of *Pasteurella multocida* strains isolated from cattle affected with haemorrhagic septicaemia. *Bull. Vet. Inst. Pulawy.* 45: 171–176.

Mustafa, A.A., Ghalib, H.W. and Shigidi, M.T. (1978). Carrier rate of *P. multocida* in a cattle herd associated with an outbreak of haemorrhagic septicaemia in the Sudan. *Br. Vet. J.* 134: 375-378.

Myint A. and Carter, G.R. (1990). Field use of a live haemorrhagic septicaemia vaccine. *Vet. Rec.* 126: 648-650.

Myint, A. and Carter, G.R. (1989). Prevention of haemorrhagic septicaemia in cattle and buffaloes with a live vaccine. *Vet. Rec.* 124: 508–509.

OIE (2000). Manual of Standards for Diagnostic tests and Vaccines.

Register, K.B., Lee, R.M. and Thomson, C. (1998). Two colour hybridization assay for simultaneous detection of *B. bronchoseptica* and toxigenic *Pasteurella multocida* from swine. *J. Clin. Microbiol.* 36 : 3342-3346.

Rimler R.B. and Wilson K.R. (1994) Re-examination of *Pasteurella multocida* serotypes that caused haemorrhagic septicaemia in North America. *Vet. Rec.* 134: 256-257.

Rimler, R.B. and Wilson K.R. (1994). Re-examination of *Pasteurella multocida* serotypes that caused haemorrhagic septicaemia in North America. *Vet. Rec.* 134 : 256-261.

Sheikh M.A., Yagoob T., Baig M.S., Mahamood. Afzal U. and Shakoori A.R. (1994) The epidemiology of haem-orrhagic septicaemia of buffaloes in Pakistan. *Buffalo J.* 10: 229–236.

Sheikh, M.A., Yagoob, T., Baig M.S., Mahamood Afzal U. and Shakoori, A.R. (1994). The epidemiology of haemorrhagic septicaemia of buffaloes in Pakistan. *Buffalo J.* 10: 229–236.

Singh, V.P., Kumar, A.A., Srivastava, S.K. and Rathore, B.S. (1996). Significance of HS in India. International Workshop on diagnosis and control of HS. Bali, Indonesia, Indonesian Department of Agriculture, 28-30 May, 1999, p 16.

Singh, V.P., Sinha, D.K., Gupta, S.K. and Chauhan, R.S. (2008). Prevalence of HS in India. Vth Annual Meet on Haemorrhagic Septicaemia at Guwahati, 5-6th September, 2008.

Townsend, K.M., Boyce, J.D., Chung, J.Y., Frost, A.J. and Adler, B. (2001): Genetic organization of *Pasteurella multocida* cap loci and development of a multiplex capsular PCR typing system. *J. Clin. Microbiol.* 39: 924-929.

Townsend, K.M., Dawkins, H.J. and Papadimitrious, J.M.(1997): Analysis of haemorrhagic septicaemia causing isolates of *Pasteurella multocida* by ribotyping and field alternation gel electrophoresis (FAGE). *Vet. Microbiol.* **72:** 69- 78.

Townsend, K.M., Frost, A.J., Lee, C.W., Papadimitrious, J.M. and Dawkins, H.J.S. (1998). Development of PCR for species and type specific identification of *Pasteurella multocida* isolate. *J. Clin. Microbiol.* 36: 1096- 19.

Townsend, K.M., Hanh, T.X., O'Boyle, D., Wilkie, I., Phan, T.T., Wijewardana, T.G., Trung, N.T. and Frost, A.J. (2000). PCR detection and analysis of *Pasteurella multocida* from the tonsils of slaughtered pigs in Vietnam. *Vet. Microbiol.* **72** : 69-78.

Verma, R. and Jaiswal, T.N. (1998): Haemorrhagic septicaemia vaccines. *Vaccine.* **16:** 1184–1192.

Zhao, G., Pihoan, C., Murtaugh, M.P. and Molitor, T.W. (1992): Use of restriction endonuclease analysis and ribotyping to study edpidemiology of *Pasteurella multocida* in closed swine herds. *Infect. Immunol.* **60:** 1401-1405.

❑❑❑

16

Leptospirosis

Synonyms : Weil's disease, Stuttgart disease, Infectious jaundice, Haemoglobinuria, Rice field worker's disease, Swine handler's disease, Sugarcane worker's disease, Canine typhus

Leptospirosis is a worldwide zoonosis. According to the occupational groups involved and the nature of the disease presentations, different names have been used, e.g. seven-day fever found commonly in Japan, Cane cutter's disease in Australia, Rice field Leptospirosis in Indonesia and Fort Bragg fever, which appeared as an outbreak in the US. Weil's disease, which is one of the severe forms of this disease, occurs in many countries, including India and other South-East Asian Countries, China, continental Europe and England. Leptospirosis exists in all the five inhabited continents and in a large number of countries. It occurs in tropical, subtropical and temperate zones. Leptospirosis is also an important cause of abortions, stillbirths and reproductive failures in cattle and pigs. Periodic ophthalmia in horse is commonly associated with leptospiral infections. Leptospirosis was first recognized in humans in 1886 by Weil and characterized by icterus. Leptospira have been isolated from a variety of animal species and humans manifesting various clinical syndromes such as mud fever and swine herd disease.

Etiology: The etiologic agent of leptospirosis is *Leptospira interrogans*. It is a thin spiral organism 0.1mm x 6 -20mm, with tightly set coils, and it is characterized by very active motility, by rotating ("spinning") and bending. Usually one or both ends of this single-cell organism are bent or hooked, but straight forms also occur that rotate and travel more slowly than hooked forms. The cells have pointed ends, either or both of which are usually bent into a distinctive hook. Two axial filaments (periplasmic flagella) with polar insertions are located in the periplasmic space. The structure of the flagellar proteins is complex. Leptospires exhibit two distinct forms of movement, translational and nontranslational. Morphologically, all leptospires are indistinguishable, but the morphology of individual isolates varies with subculture in vitro and can be restored by passage in hamsters. Leptospires have a typical double membrane structure in common with other spirochetes, in which the cytoplasmic membrane and peptidoglycan cell wall are closely associated and are overlain by an outer membrane. Leptospiral lipopolysaccharide has a composition similar to that of other Gram-negative bacteria, but has lower endotoxic activity. Leptospires may be stained using carbol fuchsin counterstain. Leptospires are obligate aerobes with an optimum growth temperature of 28 to 30°C. They produce both catalase and oxidase. They grow in simple media enriched with vitamins (vitamins B2 and B12 are growth factors), long-chain fatty acids, and ammonium salts . Long-chain fatty acids are utilized as the sole carbon source and are metabolized by B-oxidation. Because of their narrow diameter, the leptospires are best visualized by dark-field illumination or phase contrast microscopy and they do not stain readily with aniline dyes. The free living *(L. biflexa)* and parasitic leptospires *(L. interrogans)* are morphologically indistinguishable.

Cultural characteristics: Leptospires are obligate aerobes. When cultivated in a suitable aerated medium at 30°C and an optimal pH of 7.2 to 7.6 their generation time varies from 7 to 12 hours and yields are 6 to 8 x 10^9 cells/ml. Vitamins B1 and B12, and long chain fatty acids, are the only organic compounds required for their growth. Fatty acids are their main source of energy and carbon and are also required as a source of cellular lipids, since *leptospira* cannot synthesize fatty acids *de novo.* Owing to the inherent toxicity of free fatty acids, these must be supplied to the leptospires either bound to albumin or in a non-toxic esterified form. Carbohydrates are not a suitable source of energy or carbon. Ammonium salts are an effective source of cellular nitrogen. Leptospires incorporate purine bases, but not pyrimidine bases, into their nucleic acids. Because of this they are resistant to the antibacterial activity of the pyrimidine analogue, 5-fluorouracil. This compound is used in selective media for the isolation of leptospires from contaminated sources. The types of media used for the isolation and cultivation of leptospires are media enriched with rabbit serum or bovine serum albumin (BSA) and protein-free media. Liquid media are necessary for growing the cultures for serological diagnosis of infection and for typing the isolates. Liquid media are converted to a semisolid form by the incorporation of 0.2% agar and to the solid form by the addition of 1% agar. Growth is readily initiated in these media and is easily visualized as one or more rings of dense growth several mm to cm below the surface of the medium, although a lack of rings of growth does not necessarily mean an absence of leptospires. Solid media are useful for cloning the strains and for isolating leptospires from contaminated sources. Colonies in 1% agar are subsurface and become visible within 7 to 14 days. Isolates are differentiated from non-pathogenic leptospires by their more fastidious requirements, inability to grow at 13°C and susceptibility to 8- azaguanine.

Table 1. Media used for cultivating leptospira.

Nature of the media	Serum enriched	Serum replaced by albumin and tween	Chemically defined medium
Liquid	Korthof's	EMJH, PLM-5,	Shenberg's, Vogel and Hunter
	Stuart's	Leptospira 5x,	
	Vervoort's	Protein free media	
Semisolid	Fletcher's	Semisolid EMJH	
	Noguchi's		
Solid	Cox's		
	Korthof's		

Pathogenesis : The most frequent sources of infection are urine, surface water, mud and soil. Leptospires are presumed to enter via small abrasions or other breaches of the surface integument. They may also enter directly into the bloodstream or lymphatic system via the conjunctiva, the genital tract in some animals, the nasopharyngeal mucosa, the lungs following inhalation of aerosols, or through an invasion of the placenta from the mother to the foetus at any stage of pregnancy in mammals. It is unlikely that penetration of intact skin or other mucosal surfaces occurs. Drinking or inhalation of contaminated water following immersion can also cause leptospirosis. Pathogenic leptospira rapidly invade the bloodstream after penetrating skin or mucous membranes. The primary lesion in leptospirosis is disruption of the integrity of the cell membrane of the endothelial cells lining of small blood vessels in all parts of the body. Capillary leakage and hemorrhages result. These effects can be attributed to the action of a glycoprotein (GLP) toxin of leptospires. Widespread petechial hemorrhages are apparent in all organs and tissues, particularly the lungs, omentum and pericardium. Ischaemia from damage to blood vessels in the renal cortex leads to renal tubular necrosis, particularly of the proximal convoluted tubules. The resulting anatomical damage causes renal failure that can be fatal. Liver cell necrosis caused by ischaemia and destruction of hepatic architecture leads to the characteristic jaundice of the severe type of leptospirosis. Blood clotting mechanisms are affected by liver failure, aggravating the hemorrhagic tendencies. There may also be thrombocytopenia. Leptospires enter the cerebrospinal fluid (CSF) in the early septicemia phase of the illness, but there is little evidence of inflammatory response in the CSF. The anterior chamber of the eye is invaded by leptospires during acute infection, but they are trapped there and cannot move out after the local vasodilation and inflammation subside. Antibodies from circulation can enter and cause an acute hypersensitivity uveitis. Leptospires are able to persist in some anatomically localized and immunologically privileged sites, after antibodies and phagocytes have cleaved leptospires from all other sites. The most significant site of persistence is the renal tubule. Leptospires appear in the kidney 2 to 4 weeks after an acute infection, attached to an interdigitated area in the brush border of proximal renal tubular epithelium. The type of reaction in the tissues ranges from none at all to heavy scarring; animals may excrete leptospires intermittently or regularly for periods of months or years, or for their lifetimes. However, humans do not remain carriers for long, and the urine is free of leptospires at the time of clinical recovery.

Serological classification : Prior to 1989, the genus *Leptospira* was divided into two species, *L. interrogans*, comprising all pathogenic strains, and *L. biflexa*, containing the saprophytic strains isolated from the environment. *L. biflexa* was differentiated from *L. interrogans* by the growth of the former at 13°C and growth in the presence of 8-azaguanine (225 mg/ ml) and by the failure of *L. biflexa* to form spherical cells in 1 M NaCl. Both *L. interrogans* and *L. biflexa* are divided into numerous serovars defined by agglutination after cross-absorption with homologous antigen. If more than 10% of the homologous titer remains in at least one of the two antisera on repeated testing, two strains are said to belong to different serovars. Over 60 serovars of *L. biflexa* have been recorded. Within the species *L. interrogans* over 200 serovars are recognized ; additional serovars have been isolated but have yet to be validly published. Serovars that are antigenically related have traditionally been grouped into serogroups.

Genotypic classification : The phenotypic classification of leptospires has been replaced by a genotypic one, in which a number of genomospecies include all serovars of both *L. interrogans* and *L. biflexa*. Genetic heterogeneity was demonstrated some time ago, and DNA hybridization studies led to the definition of 10 genomospecies of *Leptospira*. An additional genomospecies, *L. kirschneri*, was added later. After an extensive study of several hundred strains, workers at the Centers for Disease Control (CDC) more recently defined 16 genomospecies of *Leptospira* that included those described previously and adding five new genomospecies, one of which was named *L. alexanderi*. An additional species, *L. fainei*, has since been described, which contains a new serovar, hurstbridge.

Culture Methods : Growth of leptospires in media containing either serum or albumin plus polysorbate and in protein-free synthetic media has been described. Several liquid media containing rabbit serum have been used. The most widely used medium in current practice is based on the oleic acid-albumin medium EMJH. This medium is available commercially from several manufacturers and contains Tween 80 and bovine serum albumin. Some strains are more fastidious and require the addition of either pyruvate or rabbit serum for initial isolation. Growth of contaminants from clinical specimens can be inhibited by the addition of 5-fluorouracil. Other antibiotics have been added to media for culture of veterinary specimens, in which contamination is more likely to occur. Protein-free media have been developed for use in vaccine production. Growth of leptospires is often slow on primary isolation, and cultures are retained for up to 13 weeks before being discarded, but pure subcultures in liquid media usually grow within 10 to 14 days. Agar may be added at low concentrations (0.1 to 0.2%). In semisolid media, growth reaches a maximum density in a discrete zone beneath the surface of the medium, which becomes increasingly turbid as incubation proceeds. This growth is related to the optimum oxygen tension and is known as a Dinger's ring or disk. Leptospiral cultures may be maintained by repeated subculture or preferably by storage in semisolid agar containing hemoglobin. Long-term storage by lyophilization or -70°C is also used. Growth on media solidified with agar has been reported. Colonial morphology is dependent on agar concentration and serovar. Media can also be solidified using gellan gum. Solid media have been used for isolation of leptospires, to separate mixed cultures of leptospires, and for detection of hemolysin production.

Epidemiology : Leptospirosis is one of the most widespread zoonosis in the world. The source of infection in humans is usually either direct or indirect contact with the urine of an infected animal. The incidence is significantly higher in warm climate countries due to the longer period of survival than in temperate regions. Most of the tropical countries are developing countries with more exposure of the human population to infected animals. The disease is seasonal, with peak incidence in summer or fall in temperate regions and in rainy seasons in warm-climate regions. Transmission of leptospirosis depends on the conditions favouring the survival of the organism in the environment, number of carrier animals in a population and the length of time for which carrier animals shed leptospires. The usual portal of entry is through abrasions or cuts in the skin or via the conjunctiva; infection may also take place via intact skin after prolonged immersion in water. Inhalation of water or aerosols also may result in infection via the mucous membranes of the respiratory tract. It may also be transmitted venereally, transplacentally or conjunctival routes. Transmission is also possible through coitus or A.I. The excretion of leptospires in human urine months after recovery has been recorded. The low pH of human urine limits survival of leptospires after excretion. Transmission by sexual intercourse during convalescence has been reported. Animals, including humans, can be divided into maintenance hosts and accidental (incidental) hosts. The disease is maintained in nature by chronic infection of the renal tubules of maintenance hosts. A maintenance host is defined as a species in which infection is endemic and is usually transferred from animal to animal by direct contact. Infection is usually acquired at an early age, and the prevalence of chronic excretion in the urine increases with the age of the animal. Other animals (such as humans) may become infected by indirect contact with the maintenance host. Animals may be maintenance hosts of some serovars but incidental hosts of others, infection with which may cause severe or fatal disease. The most important maintenance hosts are small mammals, which may transfer infection to domestic farm animals, dogs, and humans. The extent to which infection is transmitted depends on many factors, including climate, population density, and the degree of contact between maintenance and accidental hosts. Different rodent species may be reservoirs of distinct serovars, but rats are generally maintenance hosts for serovars of the serogroups lcterohaemorrhagiae and Ballum, and mice are the maintenance hosts for serogroup Ballum. Rats are readily infected by a low dose of serovar, *L. icterohaemorrhagiae* and large number of organisms are shed in their urine throughout their lives. Many wildlife species such as bats, mongoose, jackals, foxes, opossums, skunks, wild boar, deer, raccoons act as maintenance hosts and transmit to the accidental hosts such as humans and domestic animals. Domestic animals are also maintenance hosts; dairy cattle may harbor serovars hardjo, pomona, and grippotyphosa; pigs may harbor pomona, tarassovi, or bratislava; sheep may harbor hardjo and pomona ; and dogs may harbor canicola. Distinct variations in maintenance hosts and the serovars they carry occur throughout the world. Accidental hosts on the other hand are fairly resistant to infection but once infected they exhibit severe clinical signs. In these hosts, the renal phase is short and interspecies transmission is inefficient. Human infections may be acquired through occupational, recreational, or a vocational exposures. Occupation is a significant risk factor for humans. Direct contact with infected animals accounts for most infections in farmers, veterinarians, abattoir workers, meat inspectors, and other occupations which require contact with animals. Indirect contact is important for sewer workers, miners, soldiers, tank cleaners, fish farmers etc. Because of the high mortality rate associated with Icterohaemorrhagiae infections, this was considered an important occupational risk group despite the very small absolute number of workers affected. Livestock farming is a major occupational risk factor throughout the world. The highest risk is associated with dairy farming and is associated with serovar hardjo. Cattle are maintenance hosts of serovar hardjo, and infection with this serovar occurs throughout the world. Many animals are seronegative carriers. After infection, leptospires localize in the kidneys and are excreted intermittently in the urine. Serovar hardjo causes outbreaks of mastitis and abortion and is found in aborted fetuses and in premature calves. In addition, hardjo has been isolated from normal fetuses, the genital tracts of pregnant cattle, vaginal discharge after calving, and the genital tract and urinary tract of cows and bulls. In Australia, Scotland and USA both serovars hardjo and pomona were demonstrated in bovine abortions, but serological evidence suggested that the incidence of hardjo infection was much higher. There is a significant risk associated with recreational exposures occurring in water sports including swimming. Survival of pathogenic leptospires in the environment is dependent on several factors, including pH, temperature, and the presence of inhibitory compounds. Under laboratory conditions, leptospires in water at room temperature remain viable for several months at pH 7.2 to 8.0, but in river water survival is shorter and is prolonged at lower temperatures. When soil was contaminated with urine from infected rats or voles, leptospires survived for approximately 2 weeks. Many sporadic cases of leptospirosis in tropical regions are acquired following a vocational exposures that occur during the activities of daily life. Many infections result from barefooted walking in damp conditions or gardening with bare hands. Dogs are a significant reservoir for human infection in many tropical countries and may be an important source of outbreaks. A number of outbreaks of leptospirosis have resulted from contamination of drinking water.

Three epidemiological patterns of leptospirosis are found. The first occurs in temperate climates where few serovars are involved and human infection almost invariably occurs by direct contact with infected animals though farming of cattle and pigs. Control by immunization of animals and/or humans is potentially possible. The second occurs in tropical wet areas, within which there are many more serovars infecting humans and animals and larger numbers of reservoir species, including rodents, farm animals, and dogs. Human exposure is not limited by occupation but results more often from the widespread environmental contamination, particularly during the rainy season. Control of rodent populations, drainage of wet areas, and occupational hygiene are all necessary for prevention of human leptospirosis. These are also the areas where large outbreaks of leptospirosis are most likely to occur following floods, hurricanes, or other disasters. The third pattern comprises rodent-borne infection in the urban environment.

Reservoir hosts : The relationship between leptospires and host are easily established between some strains of Leptospira and some animal species. Leptospira form micro colonies in the lumen of the proximal convoluted tubules of kidney without damaging the epithelium. Such animals become life long carriers of leptospires and shed 100 millions leptospires/ml of urine. These urinary shedders are the potent source of infection maintaining disease cycle in the cycle. Carnivores have acidic urine and serve as short term carriers in contrast to the herbivores having slightly alkaline urine which does not affect viability of leptospires.

The primary reservoirs of most leptospiral serovars are mammalian wildlife in most of the countries viz., USA, Australia, New Zealand. Rat (*Rattus norvegicus*) is the predominant natural carrier of leptospires chiefly Icterohaemorrhagiae in the world. In India, it is *Rattus rattus* which acts as reservoirs of several serovars such as Icterohaemorrhagiae, Javanica, Hebdomadis, Javanica, Autumnalis and Inadai.

Environmental factors : Environmental factors contribute significantly in the maintenance and spread of infection among animals and man. The organisms present in the infected urine or in other material such as aborted foetus, vaginal discharge and contaminated milk become a source of infection. The urine may mix with water and mud where leptospires may remain viable for a long time. Optimum conditions for the survival of organisms are a warm and wet environment with neutral or slightly alkaline water. Leptospira infection in tropical and subtropical countries occur throughout the year whereas in temperate regions such infections are seasonal during rainy and warm months. Flood helps dissemination of infection from one place to other. Swimming pools, open tanks and fishing tanks can be contaminated and may serve as a source of infection. Rice field workers, sugarcane workers, miners, plantation workers, veterinarians, pet owners, slaughter house workers are more exposed to infection.

Clinical sings : Cattle : Most serovars of Leptospira that infect cattle cause acute, subacute or inapparent leptospirosis. *L. Pomona* is the most common cause of acute leptospirosis characterized by fever, anorexia, malaise, leptospiuria and haemoglobinuria followed by icterus and anaemia. Cows infected with *L. Pomona* have a reduced milk yield and may abort. Calves born following this infection are weak and immature. Mastitis and accompanying agalactia referred as flabby bag are observed syndrome. All the quarters of the udder became flaccid and the milk is thick and yellowish resembling colostrum and is California milk cell test positive. The fever associated with leptospirosis may last for 1-5 days and relapses for up to 53 days in 80% cases. Subacute cases manifest fever, mild haemoglobinuria and mastitis characterized by reduced amount of thick, blood stained milk. *L. Pomona* infection of South African cattle has been the cause of abortion storms. *L. hardjo* has been recognized worldwide as cause of bovine abortion, infertility and mastitis. Affected animals show fever (41°C) for 1-5 days, depression, listlessness, drop in milk production and abortion or birth of weak, premature calves. Mastitis occurs consistently and is characterized by thick, cream coloured milk with pasty consistency or by bloody milk with normal consistency. Low conception rates often occur in *L. hardjo* infected herds.

Sheep and goats : Leptospirosis of sheep manifests in two forms : acute systemic and genital. The acture systemic disease in lambs is characterized by icterus, haemoglobinaemia, haemoglobinuria, fever and death and associated mainly with Pomona serogroup but also Hebdomadis, Ballum and Grippotyphosa serogroups. The fatal haemolytic disease may kill up to 5% lambs mainly 2-4 months old often passing red urine. *L. hardjo* infections in sheep cause agalactia, abortions, still births or birth of weak lambs. Abortions rate of up to 20% caused by Hebdomadis, Australis, Pomona and Sejroe serogroups has been reported. Goats infected with grippotyphosa show haemoglobinuria, anaemia, icterus and death. Serovars pomona, sejroe, icterohaemorrhagiae and grippotyphosa have been associated with abortions in goats.

Pigs : Leptospirosis in pigs is predominantly a chronic, asymptomatic disease characterized by abortions, infertility and the birth of premature and weak piglets. Serovars of Pomona and Tarassovi mainly but also Canicola, Hebdomadis, Icterohaemorrhagiae, Autumnalis and Australis are implicated with infertility in pigs. Natural and experimental infections by *L. canicola* cause abortions, mummification, still birth, neonatal mortality and low conception rates. *L. Bratislava* is associated with infertility and has been isolated from the genital tracts of sows and boars.

Horses : Most infections in horses by Leptospirosis are subclinical. Although most serogroups have been implicated, serogroup Australis is most commonly associated with the disease. Clinical signs are still birth, abortion from 6 months to term and premature live birth, fever and icterus and death from interstitial nephritis. Leptospiral infections in horses are commonly associated with the development of ophthalmia.

Humans : Leptospirosis occurs as two clinically recognizable syndromes. The most common syndrome is anicteric leptospirosis, a self-limited illness that occurs in 85% to 90% of the cases. There are two clearly-defined stages in anicteric leptospirosis ; the septicemic stage and the immune stage. Icteric leptospirosis, or Weil's syndrome, is a more serious, potentially fatal, syndrome and occurs in 5% to 10% of the cases. The demarcation between the septicemia stage and the immune stage is not as distinct in this syndrome. Although subclinical infection is uncommon, the results of serological testing show that it occurs in some workers who have been occupationally exposed to leptospires.

Anicteric Leptospirosis : The incubation period for leptospirosis is usually 7 to 12 days, but it can range from 2 to 20 days. The onset of anicteric leptospirosis is abrupt and is characterized by fever, headache, severe myalgia, chills with rigors, prostration and sometimes, circulatory collapse. The septicemic (or first) phase lasts for 3 to 7 days. Fever is high and remitting. Headache is intense, unremitting and possibly throbbing. Anorexia, nausea, vomiting and abdominal pain occur in most patients. The most common physical finding is conjunctival suffusion in the absence of purulent discharge. Other signs include masculopapular skin rash, pharyngeal injection, lymphadenopathy, splenomegaly, hepatomegaly, and muscle tenderness. The symptoms are prominent for 4 to 7 days during the septicemic stage, at which time defervescence due to lysis occurs. Leptospires can be isolated from the blood and the CSF during this phase. The immune (or second) stage of anicteric leptospirosis is preceded by a one to three-day asymptomatic period. The onset of the immune stage coincides with the appearance of IgM antibodies. Fever, headache and vomiting are less severe at the onset of the immune stage than during the septicemic stage. The duration of the immune stage ranges from 4 to 30 days, and the leptospires are cleared from the blood and the CSF after the first days of this stage. Leptospiruria develops and persists for 1 to 3 weeks. Aseptic meningitis is the hallmark of the immune stage. Mild pleocytosis is present, with or without meningeal signs and symptoms. The CSF cell count is $<500/mm^3$ in most cases. Polymorphonuclear cells may predominate early in the illness, but mononuclear cells predominate later. The CSF protein levels ranges from < 40mg/dl (normal) to 300 mg/dl and the CSF glucose concentration is generally normal. Uveitis, iritis, iridocyclitis and chorioretinitis may also appear during the immune stage.

Icteric Leptospirosis : Icteric leptospirosis or Weil's syndrome is a form of disease characterized by symptoms of hepatic, renal and vascular dysfunction. The clinical manifestations vary in terms of severity and symptomatology. Some patients with jaundice may have no renal manifestation. Supportive therapy has reduced mortality to between 5% and 10%. Any serotype of *L. interrogans* may cause icteric leptospirosis. During the leptospiraemic phase of icteric leptospirosis, the symptoms do not suggest leptospirosis until the third to seventh day of illness, when jaundice and azotaemia develops. The biphasic course of the disease is obscured by severe and persistent fever, jaundice and azotaemia. Jaundice appears, but there is no evidence of hepatocellular destruction. Hepatic dysfunction occurs, but it resolves and it is rarely the cause of death. The serum bilirubin level is usually <20 mg/dl, but can be as high as 60mg/ dl to 80mg/dl. Hypoprothrombinemia occurs in a minority of patients and responds to administration of Vitamin K. Serum transaminase levels are mildly elevated, rarely exceeding 100U/L to 200U/L. Serum bilirubin levels peak within seven days and the increase persists for a few days to several weeks.

Renal involvement is common in both anicteric and icteric leptospirosis, but symptoms are present only in patients with icteric disease. Azotemia, oliguria and anuria commonly occur during the second week of illness, but may appear as early as 3 to 4 days after onset. Blood urea nitrogen levels are below 100mg/ dl in most cases, but may occasionally exceed 300mg/dl. Serum creatinine levels are usually 2mg/dl to 8mg/dl, although they may reach 18mg/dl. Results of urinalysis are abnormal in 70% to 80% of cases; proteinuria, hyaline or granular casts, hematuria and pyuria are typical findings. The onset of anuria is a poor prognostic sign and diuresis usually signals resolution. Hypotension due to vascular collapse occurs only in patients with icteric leptospirosis, hemorrhage occurs only in severe cases, congestive heart failure occurs rarely but non-specific ECG changes are observed in most patients. Other laboratory abnormalities include anemia, thrombocytopenia, leucocytosis with neutrophilia and an increase in the level of creatinine phosphokinase.

Pathology : Leptospirosis is characterized by the development of vasculitis, endothelial damage, and inflammatory infiltrates composed of monocytic cells, plasma cells, histiocytes, and neutrophils. On gross examination, petechial hemorrhages are common and may be extensive, and organs are often discolored due to the degree of icterus. The histopathology is most marked in the liver, kidneys, heart, and lungs, but other organs may also be affected according to the severity of the individual infection. The overall structure of the liver is not significantly disrupted, but there may be intrahepatic cholestasis. Hypertrophy and hyperplasia of Kupffer cells and erythrophagocytosis has been reported. In the kidneys, interstitial nephritis accompanied by an intense cellular infiltration composed of neutrophils and monocytes is noticed. Leptospires can be seen within the renal tubules. By electron microscopy, the tubular cell brush borders are denuded, the tubular basement membrane is thickened, and tubular cells exhibit mitochondrial depletion. In addition, minor changes are seen in the glomeruli, suggesting an anatomical basis for proteinuria in leptospirosis. Pathological findings in the heart include interstitial myocarditis with infiltration of predominantly lymphocytes and plasma cells, petechial hemorrhages (particularly in the epicardium), mononuclear infiltration in the epicardium, pericardial effusions, and coronary arteritis. In the lungs, pulmonary congestion and hemorrhage are common and infiltration of alveolar spaces by monocytes and neutrophils occurs. Hyaline membrane formation may occur. Leptospires may be seen within endothelial cells in interalveolar septa, and attached to capillary endothelial cells. In skeletal muscles, particularly of the leg, focal necrosis of isolated muscle fibers occurs, with infiltration of histiocytes, neutrophils, and plasma cells. This evidence of myositis correlates with the intense myalgia reported by some patients. In brain, perivascular cuffing is observed.

Treatment : Treatment of leptospirosis differs depending on the severity and duration of symptoms at the time of presentation. Patients with mild, flu-like symptoms require only symptomatic treatment but further medical help if they develop jaundice. Patients who present with more severe anicteric leptospirosis will require hospital admission and close observation. If the headache is particularly severe, a lumbar puncture usually produces a dramatic improvement. The management of icteric leptospirosis requires admission of the patient to the intensive care unit initially. Patients with prerenal azotemia can be rehydrated initially while their renal function is observed, but patients in acute renal failure require dialysis as a matter of urgency. This is accomplished satisfactorily by peritoneal dialysis . Cardiac monitoring is also desirable during the first few days after admission. Specific antibiotic treatment was reported soon after penicillin became available, with mixed results. Doxycycline (100 mg twice a day for 7 days) was shown to reduce the duration and severity of illness in anicteric leptospirosis by an average of 2 days.

Diagnosis : Serology on paired serum samples collected during the acute and convalescent phases of the disease is essential in confirming a diagnosis of leptospirosis. A rising titer to a specific serovar indicates infection with that of specific serovar. However, administration of antibiotic which suppress the development of antibodies, previous vaccination and prevalence of significant antibody levels in endemic areas limit the usefulness of serology in individual animals. Serological tests are useful for screening herds with a history of abortions or reproductive problems. The antibody titer declines in the dams after abortions and some mature animals do not respond serologically despite being infected. The microscpic agglutination test (MAT) with live antigens is the standard serological tests however, it requires the maintenance of live cultures of Leptospira posing health hazard to individuals. Further, it is effective on a herd basis. The ELISA test has also been used with success particularly in differentiating between acute and chronic infections. It is an alternative test to

MAT but it reacts positively at a later stage of infection (25 as compared to 10 days) and useful for screening large number of sera.

1. **Isolation of organisms :** The isolation of the causative agent and histological examination of tissues for leptospires are of major importance. As leptospires are fastidious slow growing organisms, isolation of organisms for diagnostic purpose has not been routinely relied upon. EMJH medium is used for isolating the organisms from blood, CSF and milk, aborted material, uterine discharge and tissue collected on autopsy in acute cases and urine from acute or carrier animals. At necropsy specimens should be taken from kidneys, liver, lungs, brain, body fluids of foetus, neonates and adult animals. The kidneys are the organs of choice in chronically infected or carrier animals. All samples submitted for isolation of leptospira must be kept at 4oC and sent to the labs within 3 h. Leptospira can be isolated from frozen (-15oC) specimens also. As long as 6 weeks incubation may be required for organisms to grow.

2. **Demonstration of Leptospires :** Clinical material viz., urine, foetal tissues, blood etc collected from the infected animals can be directly visualized under dark field microscope for the presence of long, motile coiled leptospires. The material may be centrifuged and stained using silver impregnation technique of Fontana and viewed. Besides, immunofluorescent technique and sandwich ELISA may be used for detection of antigens in infected animals. Immunoperoxidase staining can be sued for detection in frozen tissues. Silver impregnation technique such as modification of the Warthin-Starry method for the demonstration of spirochaetes in tissue sections are of greater value in acute than in chronic cases.

3. **Polymerase chain reaction :** It is an in vitro method for selectively amplifying target DNA sequence by more than 10^6 fold. Thus DNA of Leptospira cells present in clinical samples in a small concentration (1-10 cells/ml) may be detected after amplification either by gel electrophoresis or DNA-DNA hybridization with a suitable probe. It has the advantage that the isolation and culturing of leptospires is not required and found to be more sensitive than cultural isolation.

Differential diagnosis : In cattle, haemolytic syndrome of leptospirosis should be differentiated from babesiosis and anaplasmosis and other causes of haemolytic anaemia. Other causes of abortions, still birth, neonatal deaths and/or infertility in cattle include brucellosis, campylobacteriosis, chlamydiosis and trichomonosis and should be differentiated. The abortions, still births and mummification caused by porcine parvovirus, other viral infections, *E. coli*, mycotoxins can be confused with leptospirosis.

Control : The preventive and control of leptospirosis in domestic animals require the use of a variety of procedures. With the widespread distribution of leptospires in wildlife and the presence of a number of long term carriers, control in animals and man is difficult to achieve.

1. Control of sources in animals

(a) Rodent control : The control of rodent population by Zinc phosphide is proved to be an effective measure. The animal sheds should be covered with wirenets to deny access of rats, raccoons, bandicoots etc. The animal food should be stored in metal or concrete tanks to prevent access of rodents. The agricultural fields can be treated with calcium cyanamide.

(b) Carriers : Urine of large animals such as pigs, cattle and dogs should be examined periodically as they shed organisms for long periods following recovery. Such urinary shedders should be kept in isolation and treated if possible.

(c) Slaughter : The animals which continue to carry the organisms in the urine should preferably be slaughtered and buried or burnt.

(d) Use of protective clothing : Since leptospirosis is chiefly an occupational hazard all those persons directly involved with animals or its environment should use gum boots, gloves, aprons etc.

2. Control of infection in animals

(a) Isolation : The diseased animals should be isolated for 2 weeks and premises, tool etc should be thoroughly disinfected. Animals with temperature should be segregated and tested thoroughly. New animals should be mixed after quarantine. Penicillins are the antibiotic of choice.

(b) Chemotherapy : Leptospiric domestic animals which shed enormous number of organisms into the environment present a danger to other and should be treated with dihydrostreptomycin (25mg/kg body wt) every second day for 3 to 5 days. Abortion storms in cows and sows as well as the renal carrier state may be arrested by single treatment of 25mg/kg body wt dihydrostreptomycin when infection is due to *L. Pomona* but not due to hardjo. Chlortetracycline at 400-800 g /1016 kg for 10 days in feed reduces but not eliminate the number of carriers. New stock must be kept in isolation for 2 weeks and should be given single parenteral treatment with dihydrostreptomycin in order to eliminate a possible renal carrier state. Preventive antibiotic therapy is useful in cattle and swine.

(c) Slaughter : The animals which continue to carry the organisms in the urine should preferably be slaughtered or buried and burnt.

(d) Use of protective clothing : Since leptospirosis is chiefly an occupational hazard all those persons directly involved with animals or its environment should use gum boots, gloves, aprons etc.

3. Control of transmission

(a) Disinfection of water – The drinking water should be microbiologically safe as leptospires can survive the water if contaminated. $KMnO_4$ can be used. Village ponds should be checked for leptospires and disinfected.

(b) Hygienic measures – The animal premises should be disinfected with sodium hypochlorite to kill the organisms. Water can be made usable by addition of 0.1% $CaCl_2$ or 0.1% NaOH.

4. Education of the professional groups

The education of farmers, veterinarians, medical practitioners etc should be updated with knowledge of leptospirosis mainly in the area of diagnostic methods, mode of transmission and control measures.

5. Immunization

Vaccination is the only reliable means of controlling leptospirosis in all species. A wide range of bacterins are available for use in farm animals. Vaccines prepared with serovars prevalent in an area have been shown to be effective in preventing the disease in susceptible animals. A wide range of bacterins are available for use in farm animals. These are mostly multivalent as immunity is serovar specific and species specific vaccines are produced which include the important serovars for each species. Some vaccines do not prevent renal colonization and may promote development of carriers. The initial vaccination regimen has been inoculation of 2 doses administered 4 weeks apart followed by annual booster immunization. The vaccination schedule remains unchanged with polyvalent vaccines. In an open herd, revaccination every 6 months is advised. During episodes of clinical leptospirosis vaccination along with the antibiotic therapy is useful.

Immunity to leptospirosis is largely humoral and is relatively serovar specific. Thus, immunization protects against disease caused by the homologous serovar or antigenically similar serovars only. Vaccines must therefore contain serovars representative of those present in the population to be immunized. Immunization has been widely used for many years as a means of inducing immunity in animals and humans, with limited success. Early vaccines were composed of suspensions of killed leptospires cultured in serum-containing medium, and side effects were common. Modern vaccines prepared using protein-free medium are generally without such adverse effects. In developed countries, pigs and cattle are widely immunized, as are domestic dogs, but in most developing countries, vaccines which contain the locally relevant serovars are not available. Most vaccines require booster doses at yearly intervals. Most bovine and porcine vaccines contain serovars hardjo and pomona; in North America, commercial vaccines also contain serovars canicola, grippotyphosa, and icterohaemorrhagiae. Protection against hardjo infection has been suboptimal, but one vaccine has recently been shown to offer good protection and induces a cell mediated immune response. Canine vaccines generally contain serovars canicola and icterohaemorrhagiae. Vaccines protect against disease and renal shedding under experimental conditions, but transmission of serovar icterohaemorrhagiae from immunized dogs to humans has been reported. Moreover, immunized dogs may be infected with serovars other than those contained in commercial vaccines. A vaccine has been released recently which includes serovars grippotyphosa and pomona in addition to the traditional vaccine strains, in response to the increasing incidence of canine infection with these serovars. Human vaccines have not been applied widely in Western countries. Immunization with polyvalent vaccines has been practiced in the Far East, where large numbers of cases occur in rice field workers, such as in China and Japan. In France, a monovalent vaccine containing only serovar icterohaemorrhagiae is licensed for human use. A vaccine containing serovars canicola, icterohaemorrhagiae, and pomona has been developed recently in Cuba.

References

Angelo, P. and Brendo, A. (1998). Macroscopic agglutination test for rapid diagnosis of human Leptospirosis. *J. Clin. Microbiol.* 36(11): 3138-3142.

Antoniadis, A., S. Alexiou-Daniel, Fidani, L. and Bautz, E. F. K. (1995).Comparison of the clinical and serologic diagnosis of haemorrhagic fever with renal syndrome (HFRS) and leptospirosis. *Eur. J. Epidemiol.* 11: 91–92.

Appassakij, H., Silpapojakul, K., Wansit, R. and Woodtayakorn, J. (1995). Evaluation of the immunofluorescent antibody test for the diagnosis of human leptospirosis. *Am. J. Trop. Med. Hyg.* 52: 340–343.

Arimitsu, Y., Fukumura, K. and Shintaki. Y. (1989). Distribution of leptospirosis among stray dogs in the Okinawa Islands, Japan: comparison of the microcapsule and microscopic agglutination tests. *Br. Vet. J.* 145: 473–477.

Arimitsu, Y., Kmety, E., Ananyina,Y., Baranton, G., Ferguson, I. R., Smythe, L. and Terpstra, W. J. (1994). Evaluation of the one-point microcapsule agglutination test for diagnosis of leptospirosis. *Bull. WHO.* 72: 395–399.

Arimitsu, Y., Kobayashi, S., Akama, K. and Matuhasi, T. (1982). Development of a simple serological method for diagnosing leptospirosis: a microcapsule agglutination test. *J. Clin. Microbiol.* 15: 835–841.

Arimitsu, Y., Matuhasi, T., Kobayashi, S., Sato, T. and Cui, J. J. (1987). Serodiagnosis of leptospirosis in China by the one-point MCA method. *Epidemiol. Infect.* 99: 393–398.

Awad-Masalmeh, A. and Willinger, H. (1983). Evaluation of 2-mercaptoethanol treatment in serodiagnosis of swine leptoispirosis. *Microbiologica.* 6:133–143.

Babudieri, B. (1958). Animal reservoirs of leptospirosis. *Ann. N.Y. Acad. Sci.* 70: 393–413.

Baburaj, P., Nandakumar, V.S. and Khanna, L.V. (2006). PCR in the diagnosis of leptospiral infection.. *J. Assoc. Phys.* 54: 339- 340.

Bahaman, A. R., Ibrahim, A. L., Stallman, N. D. and Tinniswood, R. D. (1988). The bacteriological prevalence of leptospiral infection in cattle and buffaloes in West Malaysia. *Epidemiol. Infect.* 100: 239–246.

Bal, A. E., Gravekamp, C., Hartskeerl, R. A., de Meza-Brewster, J., Korver, H. and Terpstra, W. J. (1994). Detection of leptospires in urine by PCR for early diagnosis of leptospirosis. *J. Clin. Microbiol.* 32: 1894–1898.

Banfi, E., Cinco,M., Bellini, M. and Soranzo, M. R. (1982). The role of antibodies and serum complement in the interaction between macrophages and leptospires. *J. Gen. Microbiol.* 128: 813–816.

Chaudhry, R., Premalatha, M.M. and Mohanty, S. (2002). Emerging leptospirosis, North India. *Emerging Infectious Disease.* 8 (12): 1526-1527.

Chawla, V., Trivedi, T.H. and Yeolkar (2004).Epidemic of leptospirosis- An ICU experience. *J. Assoc. Phys. India.* 32: 19-622.

Debnath, C., Pal, N.K. and Pramanik, A.K. (2005). A serological study of leptospirosis among hospitalized jaundice patients in around Kolkata. *Indian J. Med. Microbiol.* 23:68-73.

Dutta, T.K. and Christopher, M. (2005). Leptospirosis – An Overview. *J. Assoc. Phys. India.* 52: 545-551.

Gussenhoven, G.C., Hoorn Menno, A.W.G. and Goris Marga, G.A. (1997). Leptodipstick, a dipstick assay for detection of leptospira specific immunoglobulin M antibodies in human sera. *J. Clin. Microbiol.* 35(1): 92-7.

John, T.J. (2005). The prevention and control of human leptospirosis. *J. Post Grad. Med.* 57: 205-209.

Kamath, S.A. and Joshi, S.R. (2003). Re-emerging infections in urban India – Focus Leptospirosis. *J. Assoc. Phys. India.* 51: 247-248.

Karande, S., Kulkarni, H. and Kulkarni, M. (2002). Leptospirosis in children in Mumbai slums. (2002). *Indian J. Pediatrics.* 69: 855-858.

Nizamuddin, M., Tuteja, V. and Shukla, J. (2006). Early diagnosis of human leptospirosis by antigen detection in blood. *Indian J. Med. Microbiol.* 24 (4):342-345.

Patel, B.K., Gandhi, S.J. and Desai, D.C. (2006). Clinico-epidemiological aspects of leptospirosis in south Gujarat. *Indian J. Med. Microbiol* 24(4): 322-326.

Ramadas, P. (1998). Biotechnology in leptospirosis. In Round Table Conference Series. (3): 41-7.

Rao, R.S., Gupta, N. and Bhalla, P. (2003). Leptospirosis in India and the rest of the world. *Brazilian J. Infect. Dis.* 7(3) : 178-193.

Report of the Brainstorming meeting on Leptospirosis Prevention and control. Mumbai, 16- 17 February 2006. Joint Publication by Office of WHO, Representative to India, New Delhi and Regional Medical Research Centre (ICMR), WHO Collaborating Centre for Diagnosis, Research, Reference and Training in Leptospirosis.

Saikada, A.P., Divale, S. and Deshpande, P. (2005). A study of autopsy findings in 62 cases of leptospirosis in a Metropolitan city in India. *J. Post Grad Med.* 51: 169-173.

Sehgal, S.C. (1998). Emergence of leptospirosis as a public health problem. *Proceedings of the third round table conference. Series leptospirosis. Ranbaxy science foundation.* 3: 7-12.

Sehgal, S.C., Vijyachari, P. and Subramaniam, V. (1997). Evaluation of leptospira microcapsule agglutination test (MCAT) for serodiagnosis of leptospirosis. *Indian J. Med. Res.* 106: 504-7.

Sharma, S., Vijayachari, P. and Sugunan, A.P. (2006). Seroprevalence of leptospirosis among high risk population of Andaman Islands, India. *Am. J. Trop. Med. Hyg.* 74 (2) : 278-283.

Shivakumar, S. and Krishnakumar, B. (2006). Diagnosis of Leptospirosis- Role of MAT. *J. Assoc. Phys. India.* 54:338-339.

Singh, J. and Sokhey, J. (1998). Epidemiology, presentation & control of leptospirosis. *Proceedings of the third round table conference. Series- leptospirosis. Ranbaxy science foundation* 3: 17-31

Singh, S.S., Vijayachari, P. and Sinha, A. (1999). Clinical- epidemiological study of hospitalized cases of severe leptospirosis. *Indian J. Med. Res.* 109: 94-9.

Sumathi, G., Chinari, P.K.S. and Shivakumar, S. (1997). MSAT – A screening test for Leptospirosis. *Indian J. Med. Microbiol.* 15: 4-89.

Suputtamongkol, Y., Sarawish. S. and Silpasakorn, S. (1998). Microcapsule agglutination test for the diagnosis of leptospirosis in Thailand. *Ann. Trop. Med. Parasitol.* 92(7): 797-801.

Terepstra, S.R. (2003). Human Leptospirosis: *Guidelines for Diagnosis, Surveillance & Control {WHO}.*1-109.

Velineni, S.,Asuthkar, S. and Umabala, P. (2007). Serological evaluation of leptospirosis in Hyderabad, Andhra Pradesh: A retrospective hospital – based study. *Indian J. Med. Microbiol.* 25: 24-27.

W.H.O. (1999). Leptospirosis worldwide, 1999. *Wkly. Epidemiol. Rec.* 74: 237–242.

W.H.O. (2000). Leptospirosis, India: report of the investigation of a post-cyclone outbreak in Orissa, November 1999. *Wkly. Epidemiol. Rec.* 75: 217–223.

Watt, G., Alquiza Lily, M. and Padne Launena, P. (1998). The rapid diagnosis of leptospirosis: A prospective comparison of the dot-enzyme linked immunosorbent assay and the genus specific microscopic agglutination test at different stages of illness. *J. Infect. Dis.* 157(4) : 234-238.

Zuerner, R. L., Hartskeerl., van de Kemp., R. A. H. and A. E. Bal. (2000). Characterization of the *Leptospira interrogans* S10-*spc*-a operon. *FEMS Microbiol. Lett.* 182: 303–308.

17

Strangles

Synonyms : Infectious adenitis, Equine distemper

It is an acute infectious disease of equines characterized by catarrhal inflammation of the upper respiratory tract with suppuration and abscessation of the associated lymph node.

Etiology : *Strepococcus equi* subspecies equi is a Gm+ cocci that produces a -β haemolysin characterized by clear haemolysis surrounding colonies growing on blood agar. It is a biovar or genovar of *S. zooepidemicus*. Equines are very much susceptible and different genetic clones occur geographically. S. equi varies in virulence which is related to M protein and hyaluronic capsule produced. *S. equi* variant without capsule causes mild disease.

Epidemiology : It occurs in horses, donkeys and mules worldwide. Outbreaks are common in breeding farms and infection is generally introduced by new arrivals that often asymptomatic. It can affect horses of any age but morbidity rate is high in foals and weanlings. The case fatality rate is 1-2% with early treatment and 9% without any treatment.

Transmission : Nasal discharge from infected animals contaminates pasture, stalls, equipments and clothes of veterinarians and attendants and is often source of infected for susceptible horses through inhalation and ingestion. *S. equi* can survive in the environment for about 2 months. About 10-40% of horses that recover from clinical disease have persistent infection of *S. equi* in pharynx and guttural pouches for many months and act as source of infection. Clinically inapparent horses with guttural pouch emphysema may shed the organism for 3 years. As shedding of *S. equi* may be intermittent, repeated culture of nasopharyngeal swabs or use of PCR examination of guttural pouch washing may be necessary to document the carrier status. Animals that have previously had the disease are less likely to develop disease on subsequent exposure than naïve animals. However, about 25% horses that recover from the disease do not develop a protective immune response and are susceptible to reinfection. Resistance to the disease is associated with the production of serum and mucosal IgG antibody to M protein of bacteria. The presence in the nasopharynx of antibodies to M protein is thought to be important in conferring resistance to the disease. Serum IgGb antibodies specific for SeM protein which is important in the anti-phagocytic activities of *S.equi* are produced by most but not all horses during convalescence. Similarly IgA and IgGb against M protein are detectable on nasal and pharyngeal mucosa after infection but not after I/M administration of vaccines containing M protein. Antibodies to *S.equri* are passed to foals via the colostrums and confers resistance to the disease.

Pathogenesis : The virulence of *S. equi* is attributable to the presence of M proteins on the surface of the bacteria, hyaluronic acid capsule and the production of a leukocidal toxin. M proteins helps the bacteria to adhere to oral, nasal and pharyngeal tissues, invasion of pharyngeal tonsils associated lymphoid structure and evasion of the innate host immune response. *S. equi* produces two M proteins – SeM and SzPse. SeM is unique to *S. equi* and plays a dominant role in resistance of organisms to phagocytosis and interfere with the deposition of C3b on the surface of bacteria and bind fibrinogen. *S. equi* that do not produce a capsule do not induce disease although they are able to infect guttural pouches and cause seroconversion in experimental studies.

Following exposure of the oral and nasopharyngeal mucosal surfaces to *S. equi*, bacteria lodge in the pharyngeal and tonsillar lymphoid tissues and multiply rapidly. The resistance of *S. equi* to non-immune phagocytosis results in accumulation of large numbers of organisms surrounded by degenerating neutrophils. The migration of neutrophils into the lymph nodes causes swelling and abscessation and oedema in tissues. Most abscesses eventually rupture and drain and the infection resolves with the development of an effective immune response. Nasal shedding of *S. equi* begins 4-7 days after infection or 2 days after onset of fever and persists for 2-3 weeks in most horses. Death usually occurs due to pneumonia. Metastatic infection of the heart valves, brain, eyes, joints, tendon sheaths or other vital organs may occur and cause a chronic illness and eventual death.

Clinical signs : The disease is manifested as an acute disease of varying severity, chronic infection of retropharyngeal lymph nodes and guttural pouches and chronic disease associated with metastatic infection of organs distant to the upper respiratory tract. The severity of the acute disease varies with the age, immune status of the animal, size of inoculum and duration of exposure to infection.

The acute disease is characterized by mucopurulent nasal discharge and abscessation of submandibular and retropharyngeal lymph node. After an incubation period of 1-3 weeks the animals show symptoms of anorexia, fever (103-105°F), serous followed by purulent nasal discharge and severe pharyngitis and laryngitis. The febrile reaction commonly subsides in 2-3 days. The affected lymph nodes become hot, swollen and painful and discharge of thick, cream-yellow pus following rupture.

Retropharyngeal abscesses may rupture into the guttural pouches, resulting in guttural pouch emphysema which is common in persistent or carrier state. If the infection is particularly severe many other lymph nodes including pharyngeal, submaxillary, parotid and retropharyngeal nodes may abscess at the same time. Local abscesses may also occur at any point on the body surface particularly on the face and limbs.

The development of suppurative necrotic bronchopneumonia in about 20% of cases occurs due to aspiration of pus and metastatic infection of the lungs. Extension of the infection into the guttural pouches occurs as a result of rupture of retropharyngeal lymph node. Metastatic infection results in the formation of abscesses in any organ but most commonly in the lungs, mesenteric lymph nodes, liver, spleen, kidney and brain. Purpura haemorrhagica can occur as a sequela to *S. equi* infection.

Lesions : Suppuration in internal organs, especially the liver, spleen, lungs, pleura and peritoneum. There is oedema and congestion of nasal mucous membrane and abscess formation in pharyngeal and submaxillary lymph nodes.

Diagnosis : It is based on the isolation of *S. equi* from nasopharyngeal swabs and abscesses. The shedding of *S. equi* in nasal discharges begins 1- 4 days after the onset of fever and abscesses often become contaminated with *S. zooepidemicus* and *S. equisimilis.*

Differential diagnosis : It is based on the isolation of *S. equi* from nasopharyngeal swabs and abscesses. The shedding of *S. equi* in nasal discharges begins 1-4 days after the onset of fever and abscesses often become contaminated with *S. zooepidemicus* and *S. equisimilis.* It should be differentiated from glanders.

Strangles	Glanders
1. It is an acute type of disease and nasal mucosa shows inflammatory changes.	1. It is a chronic type of disease with formation of nodules ulcers or stellete on nasal mucosa.
2. Lung lesions are not of tubercle like.	2. Lung lesions are tubercle like.
3. There is no ulcer or nodule formation on skin.	3. Ulcerative nodules are formed on skin.
4. Pus material shows presence of Gm+ streptococci.	Pus material shows presence of Gm- rods.

Treatment : The specific treatment of choice for *S. equi* infection of horses is penicillin either as procaine penicillin G (22000 IU/Kg , I/V every 12 h) or K or Na Penicillin G (22000 IU/Kg I/V every 6 h). Tetracycline (6.6 mg/ Kg, I/V every 12-24 h) and Sulfonamide-trimethoprim combination (15-30 mg/

Kg orally or I/V every 12 h) may be efficacious but should only be used when penicillin can not be administered. Aminoglycosides such as Gentamycin or Amikacin and fluoroquinolones are not effective. Treatment can be made based on the clinical signs.

1. Horses with early clinical signs should be treated with penicillin for at least 5 days parenterally.
2. Horses with submandibular lymph node abscessation should be isolated and efforts should be made to aid maturation and rupture of lymph node without antibiotics.
3. Systemic antibiotic therapy with penicillin is indicated in horses with advanced signs of strangles.
4. Horses with metastatic infection require systemic penicillin therapy in combination with specific therapy for the complication.
5. Guttural pouch emphysema requires either surgical drainage or repeated flushing of the affected pouch through the pharyngeal openings.

Control : Followings measures should be taken to control the disease.

1. Infected animals should be isolated immediately.
2. All the sources of fomites should be thoroughly cleaned and disinfected and bedding burned. Disinfection with phenolic compounds is preferred because they retain their activity in the presence of organic matter unlike bleach and quaternary ammonium compounds.
3. People who attend the affected horses should avoid contact with susceptible animals.
4. Newly introduced animals should be quarantined for 3 weeks and observed for signs of strangles.
5. Recovered animals should not be mingled with susceptible animals for several months.
6. In contact animals may be passively immunized by injecting immune serum S/C @ 200-300 ml for few days consecutively.
7. The majority of horses (75%) develop solid immunity to strangles after recovery from natural disease for up to 5 years.
8. The efficacy of vaccination of adult horses with *S. equi* bacterins I/M is controversial. It elicits an increase in the concentration of opsonizing antibodies but does not confer a high degree of resistance to natural exposure. Vaccination with an M protein commercial vaccine 3 times at 2 weeks interval reduced the attack rate by 5% in endemic areas.

On breeding farms, vaccination of mares during the last 4-6 weeks of gestation and of the foals at 2-3 months of age may reduce the incidence of the disease. The vaccines administered by the I/M route cause swelling and pain at the injection site. Foals that receive adequate high quantity colostrum from exposed or vaccinated mares are protected for 4 months.

An I/N vaccine containing avirulent live strain of *Streptococcus equi* with capsule has recently been developed with deletion of Has A and Has B. It should not be used in potentially exposed horses during an outbreak of the disease. I/M injection of the vaccine results in the formation of abscesses. The vaccine should not be administered to horses concurrently with I/M administered of other vaccine.

Further reading

Timoney, J.F. (1999). Equine strangles. *Am. Assoc. Equine Pract. Proc.* 45: 31-37.

Timoney, J.F. (1993). Strangles. *Vet. Clin. North Am.* 9: 365-374.

Sisson, S. and Grossman, J.D. (1953). Anatomy of the Domestic Animals. WB Saunders Co., Philadelphia 1953; p901.

Habel, R.E. (1975). Applied Veterinary Anatomy. Robert E. Habel, Ithaca NY, 1975, p57.

Newton, J,R., Wood, J.L.N., Dunn, K.A., De Brauwere, M.N. and Chanter, N. (1997). Naturally occurring persistent and symptomatic infection of the guttural pouches of horses with *Streptococcus equi*. *Vet. Rec.* 140**:** 84-90.

Jorm, L.R. (1991). Proceedings of the 6th International Conference on Equine Infectious Diseases, Cambridge, 1991, p39.

Jorm, L.R. (1990). Strangles in horse studs: Incidence, risk factors and effect of vaccination. *Australian Veterinary Journal.* 67: 436–439.

Newton, J.R., Verheyen K., Talbot, N.C., Timoney, J.F., Wood, J.L.N., Lakhani, K.H. and Chanter, N. (2000). Control of strangles outbreaks by isolation of guttural pouch carriers identified using PCR and culture of *Streptococcus equi*. *Equine Veterinary Journal* 32: 515-526.

18

Anthrax

Synonyms : Splenic fever, wool sorter's disease, Tarka

It is an infectious disease of livestock and worldwide in distribution. This is a zoonotic disease. It is also known as splenic fever because of enlargement of the spleen (splenomegaly).

Etiology : It is caused by a rod shaped bacteria of 4-8 µm X 1-1.2 µm known as *Bacillus anthracis.* It is non-motile, capsulated, aerobic, spore bearing and Gm+ in nature. The organisms remain in chains. It was the first pathogenic bacterium to be observed under the microscope, the first communicable disease to be transmitted by inoculation of infected blood, the first bacillus to be isolated in pure culture and shown to possess spores and the first bacterium used for preparation of an attenuated vaccine.

The capsule is polypeptide in nature being composed of a polymer of d(-) glutamic acid. Capsules are not formed under ordinary conditions of culture but only if the media contain added bicarbonate or are incubated under 10-25% CO_2. Capsules are formed in the body of an infected animal.

Spores are formed in culture or in the soil, but never in the animal body during life. Spores are formed only in the presence of O_2. Spores are central, elliptical or oval in shape. The spores are very resistant to physical and chemical agents. They have been isolated from naturally infected soil for as long as 60 years. They resist dry heat at 140°C for 1-3 h and boiling for 10 min.

Anthrax bacilli is Gm + and non-acid fast. When blood films containing anthrax bacilli are stained with polychrome methylene blue for a few seconds and examined under the microscope, an amorphous purplish material (capsule) is noticed around the bacilli called M'Fadyean's reaction. On agar plates, irregularly round colonies are formed 2-3 mm in diameter raised, dull opaque, grayish white with a frosted glass appearance. Under the low power microscope, the edge of the colony is composed of long, interlacing chain of bacilli, resembling locks of matted hair. This is called "Medusa head appearance." Virulent capsulated strains form rough colonies while avirulent or attenuated strains form smooth colonies. On gelatin stab culture, a characteristic 'inverted fir tree' appearance is seen with slow liquefaction commencing from the top.

The bacilli have got complex antigenic components. They are capsular polypeptides, somatic protein and somatic polysaccharides. Capsular polypeptides contain polyglutamic acid. Somatic protein are found in the oedema fluid of the infected animals. Somatic polysaccharides are hapten in nature. *B. anthracis* produces 3 types of toxins. The toxins are extracellular in nature. The toxins are (i) Factor I – denotes oedema toxin (ii) Factor II – denotes protective antigen and (iii) Factor III – denotes lethal factor. The capsular protein is encoded by virulence plasmid pX02 and protects bacteria from phagocytosis. A tripartite toxin composed of oedema (Factor I), lethal (Factor II) and protective antigen (Factor III) is encoded by plasmid pX01.

The protective antigen along with oedema factor constitute oedema toxin and along with lethal factor forms the lethal toxin. Protective antigen gets attached to specific receptors on eukaryotic cells and helps in the production of oedema factor or lethal factor in the cytosol.

Susceptible hosts : The disease occurs in all vertebrates but is most common in cattle and sheep and less frequent in goats and horses. Human occupy an intermediate position between this group and the relatively resistant pigs, dogs and cats. Algerian sheep are said to be resistant. Dwarf pigs are naturally resistant and it is impossible to establish disease in this species..

Distribution : It is one of the ancient disease that is worldwide in distribution. In tropical and subtropical climates with high annual rainfalls, the infection persists in the soil and frequent outbreaks are commonly encountered. In some African countries, the disease occurs every summer and during rainfall with death of a number of hippos, cape buffaloes and elephants. In temperate cool climates only sporadic outbreaks derive from soil borne infection.

Mode of transmission : Infection gains entrance to the body by ingestion, inhalation or through skin. Most animals are infected by the ingestion of contaminated food or water. Inhalation of infection is thought to be of minor importance in animals. Wool sorter's disease in humans is due to the inhalation of anthrax spores by workers in the wool and hair industries but cutaneous anthrax is much more common in these industries. Biting flies, mosquitoes, ticks and other insects have been found to harbour anthrax organisms and ability of some to transmit the infection has been demonstrated experimentally.

Pathogenesis : Anthrax organisms have got 3 factors which act synergistically. Protein antigen transport oedema factor and lethal factor to the target cells. Protein antigen and oedema factor combination produce oedema and protein antigen and lethal factor combination lead to fatal termination of hosts. The capsular antigen is responsible for the interference in opsonization and thus enhances the function of oedema and lethal factors.

Upon ingestion of the spores, it is transformed into vegetative form, move to lymph nodes followed by multiplication and entry into the blood and organs. The bacilli at this stage release toxins and thus produce damaging effect and oedema of tissues. Animal may die at this stage due to shock and acute renal failure.

Clinical signs : The incubation period ranges from 2-10 days. It appears as peracute, acute and subacute forms.

Cattle and buffaloes : Only two forms occur. Peracute form is most common and beginning of an outbreak. The animals are usually found dead without premonitory signs. The course is only 1-2 h, but fever, muscle tremor, dyspnoea and congestion of mucosa may be observed. After death blood discharge from nostrils, mouth, anus and vulva are common.

The acute form runs a course of about 48 h. The body temperature is high (107°F), the respiration is rapid and deep, mucosae congested and haemorrhagic and heart rate increased. Pregnant cows may abort. In milking cows, the yield is much reduced and the milk may be blood stained or yellow in color. Alimentary tract involvement is characterized by diarrhea and dysentery. Local oedema of the tongue and oedematous lesions in throat, perineum and flanks may occur.

Sheep and goats : Similar to cattle.

Horse : It is acute in nature. When infection is by ingestion there is spetieaemia with enteritis and colic. When it is insect mediated, hot, painful, oedematous, S/C swelling appear in throat, lower neck, floor of thorax and abdomen, prepuce and mammary gland. There is fever, dyspnoea, colic and swelling of the throat. The course of the disease is usually 48-96 h.

Pig : It may be acute or subacute. There is fever, dullness, anorexia and a characteristic oedema of the throat and face. The swellings are hot but not painful and cause obstruction to swallowing and respiration. Blood stained froth may be present at the mouth, petechial haemorrhages are present in the skin and dysentery may be present due to G.I. tract involvement. A pulmonary form of the disease in baby pigs due to inhalation of the infected dust has been reported. Lobar pneumonia and exudative pleurisy are present. The course is 12-36 h.

Human : Usually butchers, skinners, meat retailers, meat inspectors, tanners and veterinarians are affected. There is formation of malignant carbuncles and pneumonia due to involvement of skin and lungs. Occasionally diarrhea may develop due to ingestion of infected meat. Cutaneous form of anthrax is the usual manifestation in man.

Lesions : In anthrax, carcass decomposes rapidly with formation of gas and distension of abdomen. Rigor mortis is absent. Blood and blood stained fluid usually escape from the natural orifices and visible mucous membrane remain purple in colour. The blood is dark red or black in appearance due to lack of O_2. Subserous, subpericardial and subendocardial haemorrhages are commonly found. Widespread ecchymoses, blood stained serous fluid in the body cavities, severe enteritis and splenomegaly are strong indications of the presence of anthrax. The enlarged spleen is soft with a consistency like 'blackberry jam'. S/C swellings containing gelatinous material and enlargement of the local lymph nodes are features of the disease in horses and pigs. The lesions are most frequently seen in soft tissues of the neck and pharynx in these species.

Diagnosis : The tentative diagnosis is based on the characteristic clinical signs of bloody discharges from mouth, nostrils, anus etc. The infected carcass should not be opened. But for confirmatory diagnosis laboratory examinations are needed.

Laboratory examinations.

Staining : Thick blood films stained with polychrome methylene blue show the presence of large square ended blue rods in short chain with pink capsule (McFadyean's reaction) whereas Giemsa stained smear will show reddish discoloration of capsules.

Cultural examination : A loop full of suspected blood sample is to be streaked on 5% blood agar and nutrient agar plates and the plates are to be incubated aerobically for 18-24 h at 37°C. Smears of colony stained with Giemsa are examined under microscope for the presence of anthrax bacilli. In solid media positive cases will show cultural characteristics of 'medusa head appearance' and 'inverted fir tree appearance' on gelatin stab culture.

Animal inoculation : Materials like blood is collected in NSS and heated at 60°C for 30 min in order to kill the vegetative bacteria. 0.5 ml of the suspension is injected into the thigh of guinea pigs S/C. The animal will die in 36-40 h. Blood smear will reveal large number of anthrax bacilli.

Serological test (Ascoli's test) : This is a thermoprecipitation test and used for the detection of anthrax in hide and tissue. A piece of tissue is boiled in the water and extract is layered on a very narrow tube containing antianthrax serum. In positive cases, a well marked ring of precipitate will appear at the junction of two liquids within 5 min at room temperature.

FAT is also available for diagnosis of anthrax. An immunochromatographic test that has high specificity and does not give positive results in recently vaccinated cattle has been developed for diagnosis of anthrax. Immunohistochemical detection of bacilli in biopsy materials has also been developed. Besides, PCR, nested PCR and real time PCR with high sensitivity have been described for diagnosis of the disease.

Differential diagnosis : Anthrax should be differentiated from lightening stroke, electric injury, acute tympany, B.Q., H.S., acute lead poisoning, snake bite, HCN poisoning, acute leptospirosis, acute infectious anaemia and acute swine fever.

Treatment : Severely ill animals are unlikely to recover but in early stages treatment is effective. Penicillin (20,000 I.U. /Kg BW twice daily) through parenteral route or Streptomycin (8-10 g/day in two doses) I/M in cattle has been found effective. Oxytetracycline (5 mg/Kg BWt) has been shown superior to penicillin in the treatment of clinical cases. Antiserum @ 100-250 ml I/V daily for 5 days may be administered. Other antibiotics are ampicillin, erythromycin, methicillin and netilmicin. It is desirable to prolong treatment to at least 5 days to avoid any recrudescence of the disease.

Control

1. Control is achieved by preventing the introduction of infected animals.
2. The fodder from infected pasture should be destroyed.
3. As it is a reportable disease, it is to be brought to the notice of regulatory officials.
4. Destroy the dead body by deep burial with quick lime. Burial should be at least 2 meter deep with ample supply of quick lime.
5. Disinfection of premises with 5% Lysol, 10% Formalin or 3% peracetic acid.
6. Anthrax bacilli or spore may produce cutaneous abscess known as 'hide porter's disease', pneumonia known as 'wool sorter's disease' or dysentery in man.

Immunization

Following vaccines are available for use in animals against anthrax.

1. *Pasteur vaccine :* The vaccine strains are produced by cultivating the organisms at 42-43°C and the virulency is lost. Pasteur advocated the use of vaccine I and vaccine II. Vaccine I attenuated at 42-43°C could kill the mice but not guinea pigs or rabbits. The vaccine II attenuated for shorter period could kill mice and guinea pigs but not the rabbits. Vaccine II was used 10-12 days after vaccine I. The shelf life of the vaccine is only 7 days.
2. *Spore vaccine :* When virulent organisms are grown in 50% serum agar at 37°C and 30-50% CO_2 tension – a virulent colony develops from the margin of the present colony. It is seeded in nutrient agar and incubated. After 4-5 days, the growth is washed off in NSS and suspended in 50% glycerine saline to 1 million spores /ml. Dose : 1 ml in cattle sheep, goat and horse. Milk from vaccinated animals is usually discarded for 72 h.
3. Stern avirulent spore vaccine : It does not have any risk of causing

anthrax following vaccination and produce a strong immunity of 26 months in sheep and 1 year in cattle. Stern vaccine does not appear in milk nor can they be isolated from blood for 10 and 7 days respectively after vaccination. Vaccinated animals are withheld from slaughter for 45 days. Deaths due to anthrax have occurred after vaccination with a stern vaccine and may occur in goats.

Further reading

Andersen, G.L., Simchock, J.M. and Wilson, K.H. (1996). Identification of a region of genetic variability among *Bacillus anthracis* strains and related species. *J. Bacteriol.* 178: 377–384.

Beedham, R.J. Turnbull, P.C.B. and Williamson, E.D. (2001). Passive transfer of protection against *Bacillus anthracis* infection in a murine model. *Vaccine.* 19 : 31: 4409-4416.

Brumlik, M.J., Szymajda, U., Zakowska, D., Liang, X., Redkar, R.J., Patra, G. and Del Vecchio, V.G. (2001). Use of long-range repetitive element polymorphism-PCR to differentiate *Bacillus anthracis* strains. *Appl. Environ. Microbiol.* 67 : 7 : 3021-3028.

Cheung, D.T.L., Kam, K.M., Hau, K.L., Au, T.K., Marston, C.K., Gee, J.E., Popovic, T., Van Ert, M.N., Kenefic, L., Keim, P. and Hoffmaster, A.R. (2005). Characterization of a *Bacillus anthracis* isolate causing a rare case of fatal anthrax in a 2-year-old boy from Hong Kong. *J. Clin. Microbiol.* 43: 1992–1994.

Daffonchio, D., Borin, S., Frova, G., Gallo, R., Mori, E., Fani, R. and Sorlini, C. (1999). A randomly amplified polymorphic DNA marker specific for the *Bacillus cereus* group is diagnostic for *Bacillus anthracis*. *Appl. Environ. Microbiol.* 65: 1298–1303.

De Vos, V. and Turnbull, P.C.B. (2004). Anthrax. In: Coetzer, J.A.W., Thomson, G.R., Tustin, R.C. (Eds.), Infectious Diseases of Livestock, with Special Reference to Southern Africa, second ed. Oxford University Press Southern Africa, Cape Town, South Africa (chapter 153).

Dixon, T.C., Meselson, M., Guillemin, J. and Hanna, P.C. Anthrax. *N. Engl. J. Med.* 141:11: 815-826.

Erwin, J.L., DaSilva, L.M., Bavari, S., Little, S.F., Friedlander, A.M. and Chanh, T.C. (2001). Macrophage-derived cell lines do not express proinflammatory cytokines after exposure to *Bacillus anthracis* lethal toxin. *Infect. Immun.* 69 :2: 1175-1177.

Ezzell, J.W. Jr. and Welkos, S.L.(1999). The capsule of *Bacillus anthracis*, a review." J. *Appl. Microbiol.* 87 : 2 : 250-255.

Fasanella, A., Van Ert, M., Altamura, S.A., Garofolo, G., Buonavoglia, C., Leori, G., Huynh, L., Zanecki, S. and Keim, P. (2005). Molecular diversity of *Bacillus anthracis* in Italy. *J. Clin. Microbiol.* 7: 3398–3401.

Fouet, A., Smith, K.L., Keys, C., Vaissaire, J., Le Doujet, C., Levy, M., Mock, M. and Keim, P. (2002). Diversity among French *Bacillus anthracis* isolates. *J. Clin. Microbiol.* 40: 4732–4734.

Friedlander, A.M. (1999). Clinical aspects, diagnosis and treatment of anthrax. *J. Appl. Microbiol.* 87:2: 303-309.

Grindberg, L.M., Abramova, F.A., Yampolskaya, O.V., Walker, D.H. and Smith, J.H. (2001). Quantitative pathology of inhalational anthrax I: quantitative microscopic findings. *Mod. Pathol.* 14: 482–495.

Harrell, L.J., Andersen, G.L. and Wilson, K.H. (1995). Genetic variability of *Bacillus anthracis* and related species. *J. Clin. Microbiol.* 33: 1847–1850.

Henderson, I., Duggleby, C.J. and Turnbull, P.C.(1994). Differentiation of *Bacillus anthracis* from other *Bacillus cereus* group bacteria with the PCR. *Int. J. Syst. Bacteriol.* 44: 99–105.

Hoffmaster, A.R., Fitzgerald, C.C., Ribot, E., Mayer, L.W. and Popovic, T.(2002). Molecular subtyping of *Bacillus anthracis* and the 2001 bioterrorism-associated anthrax outbreak, United States. *Emerg. Infect Dis.* 8: 1111–1116.

Hugh-Jones, M.E. and De Vos, V.(2002). Anthrax and wildlife. *Rev. Sci. Tech. Off. Int. Epiz.* 21: 359–383.

Keim, P., Kalif, A., Schupp, J., Hill, K., Travis, S.E., Richmond, K., Adair, D.M., Hugh-Jones, M., Kuske, C.R. and Jackson, P.(1997). Molecular evolution and diversity in *Bacillus anthracis* as detected by amplified fragment length polymorphism markers. *J. Bacteriol.* 179: 818–824.

Keim, P., Price, L.B., Klevytska, A.M., Smith, K.L., Schupp, J.M., Okinaka, R., Jackson, P.J. and Hugh-Jones, M.E., (2000). Multiple-locus variable-number tandem repeat analysis reveals genetic relationships within *Bacillus anthracis. J. Bacteriol.* 182: 2928–2936.

Oi, Y., Patra, G., Liang, X., Williams, L.E., Rose, S., Redkar, R.J. and DelVecchio, V.G. (2001). Utilization of the rpoB gene as a specific chromosomal marker for real-time PCR detection of *Bacillus anthraci*s. *Appl. Environ. Microbiol*. 67: 8 : 3720-3727.

Price, B.M., Liner, A.L., Park, S., Leppla, S.H., Mateczun, A. and Galloway, D.R. (2001). Protection against anthrax lethal toxin challenge by genetic immunization with a plasmid encoding the lethal factor protein. *Infect. Immun*. 69 : 7 : 4509-4515.

Reuveny, S., White, M.D., Adar, Y.Y., Kafri, Y., Altboum, Z., Gozes, Y., Kobiler, D., Shafferman, A. and Velan, B. (2001). Search for correlates of protective immunity conferred by anthrax vaccine. *Infect. Immun.* 69: 5: 2888-2893.

Scholl, P.F., Bargeron, C.B., Phillips, T.F., Wong, T., Abubaker, S., Groopman, J.D., Strickland, P.T. and Benson, R.C. (2000). Immunoaffinity based phosphorescent sensor platform for the detection of bacterial spores. *Proc. Spie Int. Soc. Opt. Eng*. 3913 : 204-214.

Shangkuan, Y., Chang, Y., Yang, J., Lin, H. and Shaio, M. (2001). Molecular characterization of *Bacillus anthracis* using multiplex PCR, ERIC-PCR and RAPD. *Lett. Appl. Microbiol.* 32 : 3 : 139-145.

Singh, Y., Khanna, H., Chapra, A.P. and Mehra, V. (2001). A dominant negative mutant of *Bacillus anthracis* protective antigen inhibits anthrax toxin action in vivo. *J. Biol. Chem.* 276:25 : 22090-22094.

Strizhkov, B.N., Drobyshev, A.L., Mikhailovich, V.M. and Mirzabekov, A.D. (2000). PCR amplification on a microarray of gel-immobilized oligonucleotides: Detection of bacterial toxin- and drug-resistant genes and their mutations. *Biotechniques*. 29:4 : 844-857.

19

Paratuberculosis

Synonyms : Johne's disease, Chronic specific enteritis of cattle, Chronic bacillary dysentery

Paratuberculosis (Johne's disease), an infectious disease caused by *Mycobacterium avium* subspecies *paratuberculosis* (MAP), has been recognized as a major disease of ruminants for over a century. It is primarily a disease of domestic and wild ruminants and causes heavy economic losses in cattle, sheep and goat industry. It is spreading insidiously among animal population worldwide. Recently it has been shown that the disease is not restricted to ruminants only and the host range is expanding to cause disease in other species including Crohn's disease in humans. In India, the disease has been occurring since early 1930s in cattle, sheep and goats in almost every state. The disease in ruminants is clinically characterized by chronic intermittent profuse diarrhea, weight loss, emaciation and finally death.

Etiology : Paratuberculosis was first clearly described in 1895 by Johne and Frothingham as 'a peculiar case of tuberculosis' in a cow with chronic enteritis with thickening and corrugation of the intestinal mucosa and presence of acid fast bacilli in the lesions. Bang in 1906 named this disease as Johne's disease or pseudotuberculosis after having confirmed its non-tuberculosis nature. The disease was later designated as paratuberculosis.

The causative agent is an acid fast weakly Gram positive bacillus of 0.5 – 1.50 μm in length and requires mycobactin for its *in vitro* growth. Mycobactin, an iron chelating compound, is produced by all mycobacterial species with the exception of MAP. The characteristic colonies produced by the organism are either smooth or rough, small (1-5 mm), firm and glistening. Some strains from sheep produce yellow to orange colonies. Based on the biochemical tests, the organism is categorized as subspecies of *Mycobacterium avium* and called *Mycobacterium avium* subspecies *paratuberculosis* closely related *M. avium* subspecies *silvaticum* and *M. avium* subspecies *avium*.

Genomic DNA analysis provides the second method of classification.

Identification of insertion sequence IS 900, unique to MAP with 15-20 copies per organism and its detection by PCR has made it possible to detect the organism in the culture, tissues and faeces. A related insertion sequence (IS 901) is found in some pathogenic strains of *Mycobacterium avium avium* and *Mycobacterium avium silvaticum* but not in *Mycobacterium avium paratuberculosis*. Molecular genetic techniques that exploit ribosomal RNA (rRNA) differences are of little value for discriminating between subspecies because of relatively high conservation and low number of rRNA genes in mycobacteria. The detection of restriction fragment length polymorphisms (RFLPs) of the mycobacterial DNA by RE digestion, pulse field gel electrophoresis (PFGE) and field inversion gel electrophoresis can be used to identify the three *Mycobacterium avium* subspecies but not to discriminate between individual strains of *Mycobacterium avium paratuberculosis*. Minor strain differences within *Mycobacterium avium paratuberculosis* have been detected by means of an IS900 based hybridization probe, multilocus enzyme electrophoresis and randomly amplified polymorphic DNA (RAPD).

Susceptible hosts : Both domestic and wild ruminants are susceptible to the disease. Besides, the disease has been confirmed in camel, llama, alpaca, rat, mouse, cat, rabbit, fox, crow, badgers etc. Monogastric animals viz., horses, mules, hogs and monkeys may be infected but these animals remain asymptomatic shedders after experimental exposures with large doses of bacilli. The organism has been isolated from cases of granulomatous enteritis in human and non-human primates. In human beings, the disease is called Crohn's diseases.

Epidemiology : The disease has been spreading slowly throughout the ruminant populations in the world. Studies on prevalence based on various methods such as organism culture, the demonstration of mycobacterial DNA in faeces or tissue, gross and histopathological examination of lesions and serology have revealed evidence of infection in cattle up to 15% and 18% in U.K. and U.S.A respectively. In some areas of the U.S.A. up to 30% of the herds are infected. Mortality rates in affected herds are usually less than 1% but may be as high as 10%. Systemic studies on the prevalence of the disease in India have not been conducted. However, the disease is widely prevalent amongst cattle, buffaloes, sheep and goats. Most of the reports were based on the faecal examination or 'Johnin' skin test only. First case of Johne's disease in cattle was probably observed in Lahore or undivided India. Since then, large number of cases have been reported from every part of the country and many cattle farms have suffered heavy economic losses due to this disease. In a large scale survey in Assam during 1930s, high prevalence of Johnin reactors was observed at all Government cattle farms. During the same period, disease was also reported in goats and sheep in epidemic forms. High incidence of the disease (12-29%) in goat farm at Mukteswar in 1947-1949 and 10.7-18% in cattle and buffaloes based on faecal examination and Johnin skin test in Maharashtra and Haryana in 1985 -1987 has been reported. Different authors have reported the prevalence of the disease in various species of animals in Punjab, U.P., Karnataka, Haryana etc.

Young animals below one month of age are most susceptible but clinical disease does not usually develop in cattle until 2-5 years of age. However, in heavy infections calves as young as 12 months and adult animals exposed to infection for the first time may show clinical signs. Experimental studies have demonstrated that infection is favoured by the use of young animals and high doses of the organism. Other reported risk factors include intensive farming systems, acid soils, low dietary intake, stress related transport, lactation, parturition and immunosuppression due to bovine viral diarrhea disease. The nature of resistance is not fully understood as only 1/3rd of young animals exposed to infection becomes chronically infected. Some animals exposed to infection never develop clinical disease but become asymptomatic carrier and excrete bacilli throughout their lives. Interspecies transmission of paratuberculosis showed that infection have been produced experimentally with bovine and cervine strains in sheep, ovine strain in cattle and even with a human isolate in goats but calves are not infected with a caprine strain.

The disease is transmitted through ingestion of feed contaminated with infected faeces. Though it is a generalized infection, lesions are confined to gastrointestinal tract and mesenteric lymph nodes. The bacteria may be excreted in faeces by animals for up to 18 months before clinical signs are apparent, but shedding is particularly high (up to $5X10^{12}$ mycobacteria per day) from clinical cases. Organisms may also be excreted in the milk, semen, urine and intrauterine infections may occur. The excretion of organisms in the milk and the intrauterine infection are of epidemiological significance.

Molecular epidemiology : The MAP infection appears to be more complex and differentiation of MAP strains derived from different host and geographical regions is an essential prerequisite to understand the epidemiology of MAP and to implement strategies for the management and control of Johne's disease in livestock. Differentiation of MAP strains was not possible on biochemical, serological and morphological grounds till the advent of molecular tools. Cattle (C1-C5), sheep (S) and intermediate (I) strains have been described. Molecular characterization of pigmented and non-pigmented isolates of MAP lead to identification of two distinct types designated type I comprising the pigmented isolates (mainly found in sheep) and type II comprising the non-pigmented isolates which exhibit a very wide host range. The Indian isolates of cattle and goats analysed by PFGE showed that they are antigenically similar but different European strains indicating that the common diagnostic reagents to diagnose the disease and vaccine to control the disease in different species of animals can be possible.

Economic losses due to paratuberculosis are significant and a 1989 survey estimated \$ 1.5 billion annually in USA. Losses are due to death of clinical cases, reduced milk yield, fertility and weight gain.

Pathogenesis : After ingestion through contaminated feed and water, the organism invades the intestinal mucosa through M cells and reaches to lymphoid tissues. After uptake, organisms are subjected to the killing and degradation activities of the macrophages. The immunological spectrum in MAP infection appears to follow the patterns observed in *M. leprae, M. bovis* and *M. tuberculosis*. Activated macrophages cause stimulation and clonal expansion of T cells. Two subpopulations of helper T cells play major role in the resistance and progression of MAP infection. Th1 cell elicits strong cell mediated immune (CMI) response by releasing interferon γ (IFN- γ), interleukin-2 (IL-2) and tumor necrosis factor-γ (TNF- γ) during early preclinical stage of the disease which may last for several months to years as the bacilli remain within macrophage and microscopic granuloma called tuberculoid lesion (paucibacillary) are developed. Th2 responses occur later in the infection with the release of cytokines like IL-4, IL-5, IL-6 and IL-10 which enhance humoral immune response and inhibit T cell activity and the animals exhibit clinical signs.

Humoral immune response in paratuberculosis shows an inverse relationship with CMI response in cattle, sheep and goat. Serum antibody does not play protective role in paratuberculosis so disease progresses leading to infiltration of inflammatory cells causing thickening of intestinal wall. Intracellular mycobacteria proliferate and may disseminate within and beyond the gastrointestinal tract. These types of lesions are referred to as multibacillary or lepromatous type. The clinical cases with multibacillary lesions show high serum antibody titres and subclinical cases with paucibacillary lesions exhibit low antibody titres. Tuberculoid and lepromatous phases may be mutually exclusive or overlapping in animals.

Plasma leakage into gastrointestinal tract accounts for 11-21% of total nitrogen loss compared to 2-3% in normal cattle. There is decrease in total serum protein due to protein losing enteropathy. Animals with diarrhea remain in catabolic state while animals without diarrhea remain in anabolic state.

Clinical signs : The cardinal clinical signs of paratuberculosis in cattle are chronic progressive weight loss with chronic or intermittent diarrhea. The incubation period of the disease is very long and varies from 4 months to 15 years. Disease is more apparent in cows in 2nd or 3rd calving. Animals remain unthrifty with dry coat and without fever. Faeces is dark in colour and contain bubbles. Weight loss in ruminants is due to protein malabsorption and loss caused by oedema and cellular infiltration in the intestine. Animals pass typically homogenous, non-haemorrhagic and non-mucoid faeces. Diarrhoea was found to be a less constant feature in ovine and caprine but tended to occur when lesions extended into the large intestine and interfered with fluid resorption. Protein losses are generally reflected in low total protein and albumin concentration in the serum but globulin is usually unaffected. Oedema of the submandibular and other areas may be seen in advanced cases. In the later part of the disease, the animal becomes extremely weak and recumbent. Animal takes less food and water. The amount of fluid loss is more than the fluid intake and ultimately the animal dies.

Pathological lesions : The carcasses are extremely emaciated. The most characteristic lesions are noted in the caecum and colon (ileo-caecal valve) which are red and oedematous. The adjacent lymph nodes are swollen and oedematous. The lesions may extend anteriorly as far as duodenum and posteriorly into the rectum. The main macroscopic findings were of chronic enteritis, chronic intestinal lymphangitis and mesenteric lymphadenopathy. The intestinal mucosa was corrugated and thickened and subserosal lymphatics were prominent and dilated. There is no evidence of nodules like tuberculosis. Microscopically mucosa and submucosa of intestine are infiltrated with epitheloid cells, multinucleated giant cells, eosinophils, lymphocytes, plasma cells and acid fast organisms.

Diagnosis : Basically three methods exist for diagnosis of paratuberculosis : (1) Demonstration and identification of bacteria (MAP), (2) Demonstration of antibodies to the bacteria (MAP) and CMI response and (3) Detection of genomic DNA by molecular methods.

(1) Demonstration and identification of etiological agents :

(a) Faecal examination for detection of acid fast bacilli by Z-N staining.

(b) Tissue impression smear examination – Impression smears made from intestine and mesenteric lymph nodes followed by staining using Z-N method for detection of acid fast bacilli.

(c) Faecal and tissue culture.

(2a) Humoral immunity based methods : Complement fixation test (CFT), Agar gel immunodiffusion test (AGID), Enzyme linked immunosorbent assay (ELISA), Fluorescent antibody test (FAT), Haemagglutination inhibition test (HI test), Immunoperoxidase test (IPT), affinity purified antigen ELISA (APA-ELISA).

(2b) Cell mediated immunity (CMI) based tests: Intradermal 'Johnin' test, Lymphocyte stimulation test (LST), γ interferon assay and Lymphocyte migration inhibition test (LMIT).

(3) Molecular methods : IS 900 based PCR, DNA hybridization and immunomagnetic separation (IMS) of bacilli from clinical samples (faeces and milk) followed by PCR (IMS-PCR) is known to have more sensitivity than conventional PCR.

Treatment : Treatment of paratuberculosis often do not give encouraging result due to advanced course of the disease. However, anti-tubercular drug like Streptomycin, Gatifloxacin, Isoniazid etc may be used.

Control : Several countries developed national and regional programmes to either control paratuberculosis in dairy herds or accredit test negative herds as low risk sources of replacement cattle. These countries include USA, the Netherlands, Australia, Sweden France and Japan. In India there has been neither a national nor any regional programme to control the disease. However, following measures may be adopted to control the disease.

(1) All the animals in the enzootic area should be tested by faecal culture once in 6 months.

(2) Sheep and goats proved culturally positive should be disposed off by slaughter and positive cattle should be sent to Goshala/Gosadan.

(3) Faeces must be removed and disinfected and animal house should be treated with lime.

(4) Milk must be effectively boiled before feeding to the new born animals.

(5) Transportation of contaminated faeces should be avoided.

(6) Animals should be allowed to graze on pasture which are not infected.

(7) Movement of animal from infected areas to the non-infected zone should be restricted.

(8) Animal house and surroundings along with utensils should be thoroughly disinfected.

(9) Proper disposal of dung should be undertaken since it is the main source of infection.

(10) All the newly purchased animals should be tested before allowing them to mix with other members of the herd.

Vaccination : A variety of vaccines are available for paratuberculosis but its use as a method of control has been largely controversial. A heat killed and a live attenuated vaccine are generally used. In USA, heat killed vaccine is used only on small scale. Netherlands also uses heat killed vaccine. In some European countries live attenuated vaccines are used. The use of these vaccines results in substantial reduction of incidence of clinical disease, number of organisms shed in the faeces and economic losses due to culling of animals. The vaccine, however, does not eliminate or prevent infection because it does not offer an absolute resistance to MAP. The other disadvantage of vaccination is that it interferes with serological testing for tuberculosis and paratuberculosis. In India, vaccination against MAP in domestic livestock is not generally carried out. Several scientists are currently working on recombinant proteins specific for MAP to be used as vaccine. Early secreted protein of *M. tuberculosis* have been reported to be protective and it is worth to look for similar protein from MAP for their potential use as subunit vaccine.

Further reading :

Bauerfeind, R., Bebazzi, S., Weiss, R., Schliesser, T., Willems, H and Baljer, G. (1996). Molecular characterization of *Mycobacterium paratuberculosis* isolates from sheep, goats and cattle by hybribisation with a DNA probe to insertion element IS900. *J. Clin. Microbiol.* 34 : 1617-1621.

Carrigan, M.J. and Seaman, J.T. (1990). The pathology of Johne's disease in sheep. *Australian Vet. J.* 67 : 47-50.

Chacon, O., Bermudez, L.E. and Barletta, R.G. (2004). Johne's disease, inflammatory bowel disease and *Mybacterium paratuberculosis. Annual Rev. Microbiol.* 58 : 329-363.

Chiodini, R.J., Van Kruiningen, H.J. and Merkal, R.S. (1984). Ruminant paratuberculosis (Johne's disease) the present status and future prospects. *Cornell Veterinarian.* 74 : 218-262.

Chowdhry, C., Khan, M.A.R., Ramasa, G. and Sharma, D.R.L. (1980). Survey of bovine paratuberculosis. *Livestock Advisor.* 5 : 5-7.

Clarke, C.J. (1997). The pathology and pathogenesis of paratuberculosis in ruminants and other species. *J. Comp. Path.* 116 : 217-261.

Clarke, C.J. and Little, D. (1996). The pathology of ovine paratuberculosis : gross and histopathological changes in intestine and other tissues. *J. Comp. Path.* 114 : 419-437.

Collins, M.T. (1996). Diagnosis of paratuberculosis. *Veterinary Clinics of North America (Food Animal Practice).* 12 : 357-371.

Collins, M.T. (2003). Update on paratuberculosis : Control and zoonotic potential. *Irish Vet. J.* 57 (1) : 49-52.

Collins, M.T., Lisby, G., Moser, C., Chicks, D. and Christensen, S. (2000). Results of multiple diagnostic tests for *Mycobacterium avium* subsp. *paratuberculosis* in patients with inflammatory bowel disease and in controls. *J. Clin. Microbiol.* 38 : 4373-4381.

Cousins, D.V., Whittington, R., Marsh, I., Masters, A., Evans, R.J. and Kluver, P. (1999). Mycobacteria distinct from *Mycobacterium avium* subsp. *paratuberculosis* isolated from the faeces of ruminants posses IS 900 like sequences detectable by IS 900 polymerase chain reaction : implication for diagnosis. *Molecular and Cellular Probes.* 13 : 431-442.

Kurade, N.P., Tripathy, B.N., Rajukumar, K. and Parihar, N.S. (2004). Sequential development of histological lesions and their relationship with bacterial isolation, faecal shedding and immune responses during progressive stages of experimental infection of lambs with *Mycobacterium avium* subsp. *paratuberculosis. Vet. Path.* 41 : 378-387.

Manning, E.B.J. and Collins, M.T. (2001). *Mycobacterium avium* subsp. *paratuberculosis* : pathogen, pathogenesis and diagnosis. *Rev. Sci. Tech. Off. Int. Epiz.* 20 (1) : 133-150.

Miller, D., Ford, J., Sanderson, J., Withey, S., Tizard, M., Doran, T. and Hermon-Taylor, J. (1996). IS 900 PCR to detect *Mycobacterium paratuberculosis* in retain supplies of whole pasteurized cow's milk in England and Wales. *Appl. Environ. Microbiol.* 62 : 3446 – 3452.

Milner, A.R., Mack, W.N. and Coates, K.J. (1990). The sensitivity and specificity of a modified ELISA for the diagnosis of Johne's disease from a field trial in cattle. *Vet. Microbiol.* 25 : 193-198.

Mutharia, L.M., Moreno, W. and Raymond, M. (1997). Analysis of culture filtrate and cell wall associated antigens of *Mycobacterium paratuberculosis* with monoclonal antibodies. *Infection and Immunity.* 65 : 387-394.

Rajukumar, K., Tripathy, B.N., Kurade, N.P. and Parihar, N.S. (2001). An enzyme linked immunosorbent assay using immunoaffinity purified antigen in the diagnosis of caprine paratuberculosis and its comparison with conventional ELISAs. *Vet. Res. Comm.* 25 : 539-553.

Stevenson, K. and Sharp, J.M. (1997). The contribution of molecular biology to *Mycobacterium avium* subsp. *paratuberculosis* research. Vet. J. 153 : 269-286.

Tripathy, B.N. (2005). Paratuberculosis (Johne's disease) in cattle. *International J. Cow Science.* 1(1) : 16-26.

Tripathy, B.N., Munjal, S.K. and Paliwal, O.P. (2002). An overview of paratuberculosis (Johne's disease) in animals. *Indian J. Vet. Path.* 26 (1&2) : 1-10.

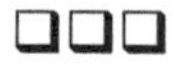

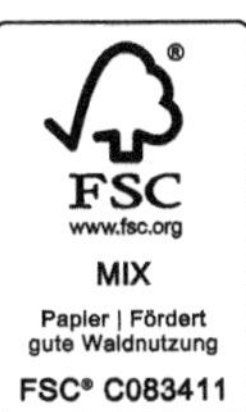

Zeitfracht Medien GmbH
Ferdinand-Jühlke-Straße 7
99095 Erfurt, Deutschland
produktsicherheit@kolibri360.de